THE MEDICINE MOTHER

A Comprehensive Guide to Holistic and Supplemental Comfort Care

DR. TEREZIA TARANTINO, DNP, RN, FNP-BC

ISBN:

DEDICATION

Philippians 4:13 reminds me, "I can do all this through Christ who strengthens me." Through you, all things are possible.

To my husband, Michael, for your unconditional love, constant support, and strength in helping me achieve my dreams. I could not do it without you.

To my children: you are all my inspiration and driving force. You motivate me daily to grow as a person, professional, and parent. I am who I am today because God blessed me with you three, opening my eyes to endless possibilities.

This book is dedicated to my mother, whose passing was the most challenging experience of my life. It inspired me to channel my grief into something meaningful—raising my children, furthering my education, and writing this book to help support other parents.

ABOUT THE AUTHOR

Terezia Tarantino was born and raised in Long Island, New York, as the eldest of four children. From a young age, she cared for her younger brothers, nurturing them as though they were her own. With a heart full of compassion, she always found joy in helping others and caring for those in need.

In 2005, while on spring break in Hawaii, Terezia experienced a life-changing accident that left her hospitalized for several days. Though the ordeal was harrowing, it proved to be a turning point, revealing her true calling and inspiring her to pursue a career in nursing.

Terezia went on to build over 15 years of nursing experience, developing a deep well of knowledge and expertise in the field. She spent many fulfilling years as an ER nurse—a role she was intensely proud of and passionate about. Her extensive experience in high-pressure, fast-paced environments has honed her clinical skills and deepened her understanding of patient care. Terezia has cultivated a unique blend of practical experience and compassionate care, making her a trusted healthcare provider.

In 2014, she married her husband, Michael, and 2018 they welcomed their first child. Terezia pursued her Family Nurse Practitioner (FNP) certification during her pregnancies with her first and second sons. Her passion for holistic medicine and supplemental care blossomed as a new mother. Motivated by a desire to keep her children safe and healthy, her knowledge and appreciation for alternative care methods grew stronger.

While expecting her third child, a daughter, Terezia returned to school to achieve her career goal of earning her Doctor of Nursing Practice (DNP). This milestone represents the culmination of her dedication to her family and her profession as she continues to make an impact in the nursing field with a focus on holistic and comprehensive care. Through her years of experience and commitment to lifelong learning, Terezia has become a well-rounded and knowledgeable healthcare provider, committed to improving the lives of her patients and their families.

TABLE OF CONTENTS

DISCLAIMER

Terezia Tarantino is a Doctor of Nursing Practice, not a medical doctor. The information in this book is intended for **informational and educational purposes only** on the topic of supplemental and comfort care. **It is not intended to replace traditional care, diagnosis, or treatment of medical conditions**. The remedies and practices discussed should complement professional medical care and are not a substitute.

Before using any remedies or implementing the suggestions provided, it is essential to consult with your trusted pediatric, primary care provider, or healthcare professional to ensure they are appropriate for your child's specific needs and health conditions. Individual responses to treatments and remedies can vary, and professional guidance is essential for making informed decisions.

In the event of a medical emergency or if your child experiences severe symptoms, please seek **immediate** medical attention by calling 911 or visiting your nearest emergency care facility. Always prioritize professional medical care and follow the advice of your healthcare provider, particularly for severe or urgent health concerns.

The author and publisher disclaim any liability for adverse effects or consequences resulting from the use or misuse of the information contained in this book. By utilizing this resource, you acknowledge that you are solely responsible for the health and well-being of your child and that this book is

NOT intended to replace medical advice or care from your licensed healthcare professionals.

Home remedies are **NOT** appropriate during instances of extremely high fevers (Those over 104), difficulty breathing, trauma (serious injury to the head, skeletal system, or deep wounds), or ingestion of poisonous or unknown substances. Always seek professional medical attention if in doubt.

> ***Always exercise caution when using hot or boiling water around children. Never leave a child unattended during steam therapy, baths, or showers. Facial steamers MAY be a safer alternative, but close supervision is essential to prevent accidental burns or injury.***

CHAPTER 01

EARS

This section is for educational purposes only. The remedies listed are intended to support comfort and wellness and should not be used as a substitute for professional medical advice. Always consult your child's healthcare provider for diagnosis and treatment.

Eustachian Tube Dysfunction (Ear Congestion)

Ear congestion refers to a sensation of fullness, blockage, or pressure in the ear, which Eustachian tube dysfunction, infections, allergies, sinus congestion, or altitude changes can cause.

Causes

- Allergies causing inflammation and mucus buildup
- Sinus infections and colds leading to congestion
- Rapid altitude changes (flying)
- Ear infections cause swelling and fluid retention
- Enlarged adenoids blocking the Eustachian tube obstructing the ear canal

Signs & Symptoms of ETD & Ear Congestion

In Infants & Toddlers:

- Fussiness or excessive crying due to ear pressure
- Difficulty feeding or refusing to nurse
- Frequent ear rubbing or pulling
- Trouble sleeping due to discomfort

Older Children may express:

- Muffled or reduced hearing
- Feeling of fullness or pressure in the ear
- Popping or crackling sounds
- Dizziness or balance disturbances
- Tinnitus (ringing in the ear)

When to Seek Medical Attention

If symptoms worsen or persist beyond two weeks, seek medical care. Immediate attention is needed if there is:

- Severe ear pain

- Prolonged high fever above 101°F (38.3°C)
- Sudden hearing loss or prolonged muffled hearing
- Pus or blood drainage from the ear

Natural Remedies for Ear Congestion:

1. *Apple Cider Vinegar & Honey Drink*

Rationale:

Apple cider vinegar has antibacterial and anti-inflammatory properties that support immune function, help clear infections, and may assist in balancing the body's pH. Combined with honey, it soothes the throat and enhances antimicrobial effects.

Instructions:

a. Mix 1 tablespoon of apple cider vinegar with 1 teaspoon of raw honey in 8 ounces of warm water.
b. Stir well and allow the child to sip slowly.
c. Offer once or twice daily during periods of congestion or illness.

Precaution:

- Not for children under 1 year due to the honey.
- Ensure the vinegar is well-diluted to avoid stomach upset.

2. *Chewing Gum or Yawning (Jaw Movement Therapy)*

Rationale:

The movement of jaw muscles stimulates the Eustachian tubes, helping them open and promoting natural fluid drainage from the middle ear. Chewing, yawning, or swallowing may help "pop" the ears and relieve built-up pressure.

Instructions:

a. Offer sugar-free chewing gum or hard candy (age appropriate) to encourage frequent swallowing.

b. Practice exaggerated yawning or encourage fake yawns to help open the Eustachian tubes.

Precaution:

- Use only with children old enough to safely chew gum or candy without choking risk.
- Supervise use and avoid gum with artificial dyes or sweeteners.

3. *Ear Massage for Drainage*

Rationale:

Gentle massage around the ear and down the neck promotes lymphatic drainage, reduces pressure, and may help open the Eustachian tubes.

Instructions:

a. Using fingertips, gently massage behind the ear and down the side of the neck in circular motions.
b. Repeat for 1–2 minutes on each side, 2–3 times daily.

Precaution:

- Avoid massaging over painful or visibly inflamed areas.
- Stop if the child complains of discomfort.

4. *Essential Oils for Decongestion*

Rationale:

Eucalyptus and peppermint oils have decongestant, anti-inflammatory, and antimicrobial properties. When used in steam or applied topically (when diluted), they help open the nasal passages and support eustachian tube drainage.

Instructions:

a. Steam Inhalation: Add 3–5 drops of eucalyptus oil to boiling water, cover the head with a towel, and inhale the steam deeply.
b. Diffusion: Add oils to a room diffuser as directed.
c. Topical Application: Mix 1–2 drops of essential oil with a carrier oil and apply gently behind the ears and along the jawline.

Precaution:

- Only use essential oils labeled safe for children and avoid direct contact with mucous membranes.
- Never leave a child unattended near boiling water or steam.
- Always perform a patch test before topical application.

5. Gargling Salt Water (Age 4+)

Rationale:

Gargling with warm salt water helps reduce throat inflammation, clear nasal drip, and indirectly relieve ear pressure by improving sinus drainage.

Instructions:

a. Mix 1 teaspoon of high-quality salt (e.g., sea salt or Himalayan salt) in a glass of warm water.
b. Have the child gargle for 30 seconds, then spit it out.
c. Repeat 2–3 times daily, especially after meals.

Precaution:

- Only use with children who can reliably gargle and spit.
- Supervise to ensure they do not swallow the solution.

6. *Heating Pad Therapy for Ear Pain & Drainage*

Rationale:
Warm compresses help dilate blood vessels, improve circulation, and loosen mucus. This can relieve ear pain and promote drainage of the middle ear and sinus passages.

Instructions:

a. Use a warm (not hot) heating pad, rice sock, or damp washcloth.
b. Place it gently over the ear and jaw area while the child lies on their side.
c. Leave for 10–20 minutes and repeat every few hours as needed.

Precaution:

- Always test temperature before applying.
- Never leave young children unattended with heating devices.

7. *Hydration*

Rationale:

Adequate fluid intake helps thin mucus, facilitating easier drainage through the sinuses and Eustachian tubes, which relieves pressure behind the ears.

Instructions:

a. Encourage the child to drink plenty of water throughout the day.
b. Offer warm broths or caffeine-free herbal teas to soothe the throat and hydrate.
c. Increase fluids during illness or if signs of congestion are present.

Precaution:

- Avoid sugary drinks and artificially flavored beverages that may increase inflammation or mucous production.

8. Manual Valsalva Maneuver (Older Children Only)

Rationale:

This technique gently forces the Eustachian tubes open by creating internal pressure, helping to equalize ear pressure and relieve fullness or popping.

Instructions:

a. Have the child take a deep breath and pinch their nose shut.
b. While keeping their mouth closed, ask them to try blowing gently through their nose.
c. A "pop" may occur, signaling the Eustachian tube has opened.

Precaution:

- Use only in children old enough to understand the technique.
- Never force the blow—excessive pressure can damage the eardrum.

9. Mullein Garlic Ear Oil

Rationale:

A blend of mullein and garlic infused in oil has natural anti-inflammatory, antibacterial, and pain-relieving properties. It supports drainage and calms irritation in the outer and middle ear.

Instructions:

a. Warm the bottle in a bowl of hot (not boiling) water.
b. Test temperature on the wrist to ensure it's safe.
c. Use a clean dropper to place 2–3 drops in the affected ear.
d. Let the child lie on their side for 5–10 minutes before draining.

Precaution:

- Do not use if there is any drainage from the ear or suspected eardrum rupture.
- Use only filtered oil preparations labeled for ear use.

10. Nasal Saline Rinse

Rationale:

Rinsing the nasal passages helps flush out allergens, irritants, and mucus that may contribute to ear congestion by blocking the Eustachian tubes.

Instructions:

a. Use a neti pot, saline spray, or nasal bulb to rinse the nostrils.
b. Perform once or twice daily, especially during congestion.

Precaution:

- Always use sterile, distilled, or previously boiled and cooled water.
- Not recommended for infants or very young children without provider guidance.

11. Olive Oil Ear Drops

Rationale:

Warm olive oil softens earwax, soothes irritated tissues, and may reduce discomfort from pressure and mild congestion.

Instructions:

a. Warm a few drops of olive oil until just lukewarm.
b. Tilt the head and place 2–3 drops into the ear.
c. Keep the head tilted for 5–10 minutes, then drain.
d. Use 1–2 times daily until relief is felt.

Precaution:

- Do not use if there is fluid drainage, ear injury, or suspected eardrum perforation.
- Always test oil temperature before use.

12. Steam Therapy

Rationale:

Steam helps moisten and loosen thick mucus in the nasal passages and Eustachian tubes. This reduces inflammation and promotes natural drainage, especially when essential oils are added.

Instructions:

a. Boil water and pour it into a heat-safe bowl.
b. Add 1–2 drops of child-safe eucalyptus or peppermint essential oil.
c. Place a towel over the child's head and have them inhale the steam for 5–10 minutes under supervision.

Precaution:

- Keep boiling water out of reach of children.
- Never leave children unsupervised during steam therapy.
- Only use essential oils labeled safe for children and age-appropriate.

Outer Ear Infection (Otitis Externa)

Otitis Externa, or **Swimmer's Ear**, is an infection or inflammation of the **outer ear canal**. It is often caused by moisture trapped in the ear, which creates an ideal environment for bacteria or fungi to grow. It typically affects school-aged children during warm months or after frequent swimming but can occur at any age.

Causes:

- Water trapped in the ear canal after swimming or bathing
- Bacterial or fungal infections (commonly *Pseudomonas* or *Aspergillus*)
- Overcleaning or irritation of the ear canal with cotton swabs
- Use of hearing aids or earbuds that damage ear lining
- Eczema or skin sensitivity inside the ear canal

Signs & Symptoms of Otitis Externa:

In Infants & Toddlers:

- Irritability or frequent crying when lying on the affected ear.
- Pulling at the ear
- Sensitivity to touch near the outer ear.
- Drainage from the ear (often clear, yellow, or pus-like)

Older Children May Communicate:

- Pain when touching or tugging the outer ear.
- Itching inside the ear canal
- Feeling of fullness or blockage
- Mild hearing loss or muffled hearing
- Swelling or redness at the ear opening

When to Seek Medical Attention:

Seek care promptly if your child experiences.

- **Worsening pain or spreading redness** around the ear or face
- **Fever over 101°F (38.3°C)**
- **Persistent discharge** or foul-smelling fluid from the ear
- **Swollen lymph nodes** near the ear or jaw
- **No improvement within 2–3 days** of home treatment

Preventative Remedies for Swimmer's Ear (otitis externa):

For kids prone to outer ear infections, these can be done each time after swimming as a preventative measure.

1. Breast Milk Drops (Infants & Toddlers)

Rationale:

Breast milk contains antibodies and immune-regulating proteins that help reduce inflammation and fight infection. Due to its soothing and antimicrobial properties, it is especially useful for exclusively breastfed infants with mild outer ear irritation.

Instructions:

a. Express a few drops of fresh breast milk into a sterile container.
b. Use a clean dropper to place 2–3 drops in the affected ear.
c. Let sit for 5–10 minutes, then allow to drain naturally.
d. Repeat 2–3 times daily as needed.

Precaution:

- Only use for infants over 6 weeks of age.
- Do not use if there is fluid or pus draining from the ear.
- Always use freshly expressed milk and discontinue if signs of irritation occur.

2. *Coconut Oil*

Rationale:
Coconut oil is naturally antibacterial, antifungal, and moisturizing, which helps soothe and protect the irritated ear canal from infection and dryness.

Instructions:

a. Warm organic virgin coconut oil until it becomes liquid, ensuring it is not hot.
b. Place 1–2 drops in the affected ear using a clean dropper.
c. Let it sit for 5 minutes, then tilt the head to allow draining.
d. Use once daily as needed to relieve discomfort.

Precaution:

- Do not use if the child has a ruptured eardrum or active drainage.
- Always test temperature before applying.

3. *Drying the Ears After Swimming or Bathing*

Rationale:

Keeping the ear canal dry helps prevent bacterial and fungal overgrowth, especially in children prone to recurrent swimmer's ear.

Instructions:

a. After swimming or bathing, tilt the head to each side to drain water from the ears.
b. Use a clean, dry towel to gently pat the outer ear.
c. If infections are recurrent, use preventive measures such as vinegar drops.
d. Consider swimmers' earplugs or a snug swim cap to reduce water entry.

Precaution:

- Avoid inserting cotton swabs or objects into the ear canal.
- Ensure ears are completely dry before bedtime if moisture is retained.

4. Garlic & Mullein Oil Drops

Rationale:

Garlic and mullein oils have antibacterial, antiviral, and anti-inflammatory properties. Garlic's allicin helps kill harmful bacteria, while mullein soothes inflamed tissue. Together, they provide a gentle yet effective remedy for outer ear irritation.

Instructions:

a. Warm the oil by placing the sealed bottle in a bowl of warm water.
b. Test the temperature on your wrist.
c. Use a clean dropper to place 2–3 drops in the ear.
d. Allow it to sit for 5–10 minutes, then drain.

Precaution:

- Do not use if there is active discharge or suspected eardrum rupture.
- Always use filtered oil; never insert raw garlic.
- Discontinue if redness or irritation occurs.

5. Hydrogen Peroxide

Rationale:

Hydrogen peroxide gently cleanses the ear canal by breaking up wax and debris. It has mild antimicrobial effects and helps remove trapped water that can lead to infection.

Instructions:

a. Mix equal parts 3% hydrogen peroxide and distilled water.

b. Place 2–3 drops in the affected ear.
c. Let it bubble for 30 seconds, then tilt the head to drain.
d. Use only once per day if needed.

Precaution:

- Do not use in children with ruptured eardrums or if pain worsens.
- Avoid overuse, as it may irritate the skin lining the ear canal.

6. *Tea Tree Oil Dilution*

Rationale:

Tea tree oil contains terpinen-4-ol, known for its strong antibacterial, antifungal, and anti-inflammatory effects. When diluted, it can help address infection and soothe irritation.

Instructions:

a. Mix 1 drop of tea tree oil with 1 teaspoon of warm carrier oil (olive or coconut).
b. Soak a clean cotton ball in the diluted oil.
c. Gently place the cotton ball at the opening of the ear without pushing it inside.
d. Leave in place for 10–15 minutes, then remove.

Precaution:

- Never use undiluted tea tree oil.
- Not recommended for children under age 2.
- Discontinue if any irritation or skin reaction occurs.

7. *Vinegar & Alcohol Ear Drops*

Rationale:

A mixture of white vinegar and rubbing alcohol restores the natural acidic balance of the ear canal and removes residual moisture. This makes the environment less favorable for bacterial and fungal growth.

Instructions:

a. Mix equal parts white vinegar and isopropyl alcohol in a clean container.
b. Place 2–3 drops in the affected ear using a sterile dropper.
c. Keep the head tilted for 30 seconds, then allow the liquid to drain.
d. Repeat 1–2 times daily if needed.

Precaution:

- Not for use if the eardrum is ruptured or if there is pain during application.
- Alcohol may sting if the skin is irritated—discontinue if discomfort occurs.

8. White Vinegar and Peroxide

Rationale:

This combination helps prevent swimmer's ear by restoring the ear canal's pH, dissolving debris, and killing bacteria and fungi. Vinegar acidifies the ear environment, while peroxide gently cleanses wax buildup.

Instructions:

a. Mix equal parts white vinegar and hydrogen peroxide.
b. Place 1–2 drops in each ear after swimming to dry and sanitize.

Precaution:

- Do not use if the ear is actively draining or injured.
- Avoid use more than once daily to prevent over-drying or irritation.

Ear Infection (Otitis Media)

Otitis Media is an **infection or inflammation of the middle ear**, the space behind the eardrum. Due to their smaller and more horizontal Eustachian tubes (which connect the middle ear to the back of the throat), ear infections are among the most common childhood illnesses, especially in infants and young children.

Causes

- Viral or bacterial infections
- Fluid buildup behind the eardrum
- Inflammation due to colds or allergies

Signs & Symptoms of Otitis Media

In Infants & Toddlers:

- Pulling at the ear
- Crying more than usual (irritability)
- Tugging, Difficulty sleeping
- Fever (may not always be present)
- Trouble hearing or responding to sounds

Older Children May Communicate:

- Ear pain or pressure
- Muffled or reduced hearing
- Dizziness or balance issues

Important Warning: Do NOT put anything in the ear if the eardrum ruptures.

If a child has symptoms of a ruptured eardrum (tympanic membrane), DO NOT put any liquids, oils, or drops into the ear. Introducing substances into the ear when the eardrum is ruptured can cause further irritation, infection, and potential damage to deeper ear structures.

Signs of a Ruptured Eardrum:

If you notice **any of these symptoms**, seek additional medical attention immediately:

- **Sudden Relief from Ear Pain**—If severe ear pain suddenly goes away, this could indicate that the eardrum has burst, releasing built-up pressure.
- **Excessive fluid or Pus Drainage from the Ear** – Clear, yellow, or bloody fluid draining from the ear can signify an infection and a rupture.
- **Hearing Loss or Muffled Hearing** – A ruptured eardrum can cause temporary hearing loss in the affected ear.
- **Ringing or Buzzing Sounds (Tinnitus)** – Some people experience a high-pitched ringing noise after the eardrum perforates.
- **Dizziness or Balance Issues** – The inner ear plays a role in balance, and a rupture may cause dizziness or vertigo.

When to Seek Medical Attention:

If symptoms **worsen or do not improve within 3 days,** or if the child has:

- Severe ear pain
- Prolonged fevers over 101°F (38.3°C)
- Swelling or redness spreading beyond the ear
- Drainage of pus or blood from the ear

Consult a doctor for further evaluation.

What to Do if You Suspect a Ruptured Eardrum:

- **Keep the ear dry** – Avoid swimming, bathing, or any moisture entering the ear.
- **Tilt the head sideways** to allow any fluid to drain naturally.

- **Cover the ear loosely** with a **clean, dry cotton ball** (do not push it inside).
- **Seek medical attention** – A healthcare provider can assess the damage and provide appropriate treatment.

Natural Remedies for Otitis Media:

1. *Breast Milk Drops (Infants & Toddlers)*

Rationale:

Breast milk contains antibodies and immune-modulating proteins that can help reduce inflammation and fight infection. It is gentle, natural, and particularly beneficial for exclusively breastfed infants experiencing mild ear irritation.

Instructions:

a. Express a few drops of fresh breast milk into a sterile container.
b. Use a clean dropper to place 2–3 drops in the affected ear.
c. Let sit for 5–10 minutes, then allow to drain naturally.
d. Repeat 2–3 times daily as needed.

Precaution:

- Only use in infants over 6 weeks old.
- Do not use if there is fluid or pus draining from the ear.
- Discontinue if irritation or redness develops.

2. *Ear Massage for Lymphatic Drainage*

Rationale:

Gentle massage helps stimulate lymphatic flow, relieve pressure in the middle ear, and reduce fluid buildup by encouraging natural drainage.

Instructions:

a. Using your fingertips, gently massage behind the ear and down the neck toward the collarbone in small circles.
b. Massage for 1–2 minutes, several times per day.
c. May be done with or without diluted essential oils such as lavender or chamomile, appropriate for the child's age.

Precaution:

- Avoid massaging over visibly swollen or painful areas.
- Discontinue if the child expresses discomfort.

3. Elevation During Sleep

Rationale:

Keeping the head elevated during sleep supports natural fluid drainage from the middle ear and can reduce nighttime pain associated with pressure buildup.

Instructions:

a. For toddlers and older children, place an extra pillow under the mattress or use a wedge.
b. For infants, use only crib-safe elevation methods and only under the guidance of a healthcare provider.

Precaution:

- Do not place pillows directly under an infant's head due to suffocation risk.
- Only elevate with pediatrician-approved methods for babies.

4. *Garlic Oil Drops*

Rationale:

Garlic oil has strong antibacterial, antiviral, and anti-inflammatory properties. Its active compound, allicin, helps fight infection, reduce inflammation, and relieve pain. When gently warmed, garlic oil can soothe symptoms and support healing.

Instructions:

a. Warm the garlic oil slightly by placing the sealed bottle in a bowl of warm (not hot) water.
b. Test the temperature on your wrist to ensure it is comfortably warm.
c. Using a clean dropper, place 2–3 drops into the affected ear while the child lies on their side.
d. Allow to sit for 5–10 minutes, then tilt the head to drain.
e. Repeat 2–3 times daily as needed.

Precaution:

- Do not use if there is suspected eardrum rupture or fluid drainage.
- Only use filtered, pre-prepared garlic oil (not raw garlic pulp).
- Discontinue if redness, rash, or irritation occurs.

5. *Olive Oil Drops*

Rationale:

Warm olive oil can help lubricate and soothe the ear canal, reduce irritation, and potentially promote drainage in cases of non-ruptured ear infections.

Instructions:

a. Warm the olive oil gently and test on your wrist to confirm safe temperature.
b. Place 2–3 drops in the affected ear with a clean dropper.

c. Have the child rest on their side for 5–10 minutes.
d. Repeat up to 3 times per day as needed.

Precaution:

- Do not use in ears with ruptured eardrums or active discharge.
- Always test temperature to avoid burns.

6. *Onion Poultice*

Rationale:

When heated, onions release sulfur compounds with antibacterial and anti-inflammatory benefits. The warmth and natural vapors can reduce ear pain and support healing.

Instructions:

a. Bake a halved onion at 350°F (175°C) for 30 minutes, until soft and steaming.
b. Let it cool to a warm (not hot) temperature.
c. Place the cut side down inside a mug to concentrate steam.
d. Hold the mug near the affected ear for 10–15 minutes.
e. Repeat 2–3 times daily for symptom relief.

Precaution:

- Test temperature to avoid burns.
- Never place the onion directly into the ear canal.
- Discontinue if skin irritation occurs.

7. *Steam Therapy*

Rationale:

Steam helps loosen mucus and promote Eustachian tube drainage, especially when congestion is a contributing factor to ear fluid buildup. Adding essential oils provides further anti-inflammatory support.

Instructions:

a. Sit in a steamy bathroom with hot water running for 10–15 minutes, especially before bedtime.
b. For older children, use a bowl of hot water with a towel over the head.
c. Add 1–2 drops of eucalyptus or lavender essential oil (age 2+ only) for added relief.

Precaution:

- Never leave a child unattended around hot water or steam.
- Ensure essential oils used are age-appropriate and safe for children.
- Do not use steam if the child has asthma or sensitivity to vapor.

8. Warm Compress

Rationale:

Applying heat increases circulation, relaxes surrounding muscles, and helps relieve ear pain by softening trapped fluid and reducing inflammation.

Instructions:

a. Soak a clean washcloth in warm water and wring it out.
b. Fold and place it gently over the affected ear for 10–15 minutes.
c. Reheat and reapply every few hours as needed for comfort.

Precaution:

- Always test the compress temperature to avoid burns.
- Do not use if the skin is broken or if there is visible irritation.

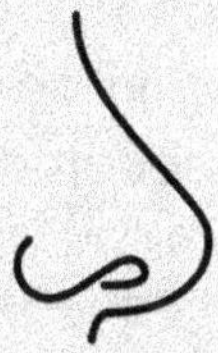

CHAPTER 02

NOSE

This section is for educational purposes only. The remedies listed are intended to support comfort and wellness and should not be used as a substitute for professional medical advice. Always consult your child's healthcare provider for diagnosis and treatment.

Nasal Congestion & Runny Nose (Rhinitis)

Rhinitis is the inflammation of the mucous membrane inside the nose, leading to symptoms such as sneezing, runny nose (rhinorrhea), nasal congestion, itching, and postnasal drip. Nasal congestion, also known as a stuffy nose, occurs when the nasal passages become swollen due to inflammation, irritation, or excess mucus.

Causes:

- Allergies
- Colds and Flu
- Weather changes
- Irritants

Signs & Symptoms of Congestion & Rhinitis:

- Stuffy or runny nose
- Sneezing & itchy nose
- Coughing
- Mouth breathing
- Snoring & sleeping issues
- Decreased appetite
- Irritability & fatigue

When to Seek Medical Attention

If symptoms worsen or persist beyond two weeks, seek medical care. Immediate attention is needed if there is:

- Persistent high fever **102°F (38.9°C)** or lasting over 3 days.
- Severe breathing difficulty, struggling to breathe (flaring nostrils or chest retractions).
- Thick green or yellow mucus with fever may indicate infection.
- Ear pain and drainage may indicate an ear infection.

- Swelling around the eyes and face
- Wheezing or a persistent cough

Natural Remedies for Congestion and Runny Nose:

1. Adequate Hydration

Rationale:

Proper fluid intake thins nasal mucus, making it easier to clear the sinuses and reduce congestion.

Instructions:

a. Offer water, breast milk, broths, or age-appropriate electrolyte fluids frequently.
b. Warm fluids such as chamomile tea (age-appropriate) may offer additional soothing effects.

Precaution:

- Avoid sugary or caffeinated drinks, which may worsen inflammation.

2. Bromelain (from Pineapple) or Supplement (Age 3+)

Rationale:

Bromelain is a natural enzyme that reduces mucus production and has mild anti-inflammatory effects in the sinuses.

Instructions:

a. Offer fresh pineapple in moderation or give a child-formulated bromelain supplement under pediatric supervision.
b. Use only as directed on pediatric-specific labels.

Precaution:

- Do not use in children with pineapple allergies or oral irritation.

3. Elderflower Tea or Tincture (Age 2+)

Rationale:

Elderflower is a gentle herb that supports sinus drainage and helps ease congestion. It also offers mild fever-reducing and anti-inflammatory effects.

Instructions:

a. Steep 1 teaspoon of dried elderflower in 1 cup of hot water for 5–10 minutes, then strain.
b. Allow to cool to a warm, safe temperature.
c. Offer ¼ to ½ cup up to twice daily during acute congestion.
d. Alternatively, use a child-safe elderflower tincture per label instructions or provider guidance.

Precaution:

- Use only age-appropriate formulations.
- Do not combine with other fever-reducing herbs without consulting a provider.

4. Essential Oil Diffusion (Age 2+)

Rationale:

Diffusing child-safe essential oils like eucalyptus or lavender helps clear nasal passages and promote calm during illness.

Instructions:

a. Add 2–3 drops of organic, child-safe essential oils to a cool mist diffuser in the child's room.
b. Run for 30–60 minutes at bedtime or during nap time.

Precution:

- Only use oils labeled safe for pediatric use.
- Keep diffuser out of reach and use in a well-ventilated area.

5. *Homemade Vapor Rub (Topical, Age 2+)*

Rationale:

This natural chest rub uses essential oils like eucalyptus and peppermint to help open nasal passages and relieve sinus pressure.

Instructions:

a. In a small jar, mix:

- ¼ cup coconut oil
- 1 tablespoon beeswax pellets
- 5 drops eucalyptus oil
- 5 drops peppermint oil (omit for children under 3)
- 3 drops lavender oil

b. Melt the beeswax and coconut oil together, remove from heat, and stir in essential oils.

c. Let cool and solidify. Apply a small amount to the chest, neck, and upper back.

Precaution:

- Do not apply to broken skin or directly under the nose.
- Avoid peppermint oil in children under 3 unless advised by a provider.
- Perform a patch test first to check for skin sensitivity.

6. *Massage & Pressure Point Techniques*

Rationale:

Gentle massage and acupressure techniques can stimulate sinus drainage, relieve pressure, and reduce facial and upper respiratory tract inflammation.

Instructions:

A. ***Eyebrow & Bridge of Nose Massage***

   a. Use your index fingers to apply gentle circular pressure between the eyebrows.
   b. Glide fingers slowly down the sides of the nose to the nostrils.
   c. Repeat 10–15 times, especially before bed.

Effect: Encourages sinus drainage and relieves upper nasal pressure.

B. ***Cheekbone Pressure Points (Maxillary Sinuses)***

   a. Place fingertips on either side of the face, just below the cheekbones.
   b. Press gently and hold for 30 seconds, then release.
   c. Repeat 3–5 times as needed.

Effect: Eases pressure and promotes drainage.

C. ***Nasal Side Sweep***

   a. Use thumbs to gently sweep from the top of the nostrils outward along the cheek.
   b. Repeat in a downward motion toward the jawline.
   c. Do this for 1–2 minutes, 2–3 times daily.

Effect: Opens nasal passages and reduces swelling.

D. ***Under-Ear Drainage Massage***

   a. Stroke gently from behind the earlobe down the neck toward the collarbone.
   b. Use rhythmic strokes for 30–60 seconds per side.

Effect: Promotes lymphatic drainage and relieves ENT congestion.

E. ***Thumb-to-Third-Eye Pressure***

   a. Apply steady pressure to the center of the forehead (between the eyebrows) for 30 seconds.
   b. Release and repeat as needed.

Effect: May reduce sinus headaches and encourage drainage.

Precaution:

- Stop if any pressure points feel tender or cause discomfort.
- Do not use oils on skin with known sensitivities unless diluted and patch tested.

7. Onion and Honey Syrup (Age 1+)

Rationale:

Onion acts as a natural expectorant, helping break down mucus, while honey soothes inflamed tissues and supports immune function.

Instructions:

a. Place thinly sliced onion in a small jar and cover with raw honey.
b. Let sit 4–6 hours or overnight until liquid is drawn out.
c. Strain and give 1 teaspoon 2–3 times daily during congestion.

Precaution:

- Do not give to children under 1 year due to risk of botulism.
- Discontinue if the child shows signs of allergy or digestive upset.

8. Peppermint Tea (Age 3+)

Rationale:

Peppermint tea contains menthol, which helps open the nasal passages, thin mucus, and ease headaches related to sinus pressure.

Instructions:

a. Steep 1 peppermint tea bag (or 1 tsp dried peppermint) in 1 cup hot water for 5–10 minutes.
b. Let cool to a safe drinking temperature.
c. Offer in small sips up to 2 times daily during active symptoms.

Precaution:

- Do not offer to children under 3.
- Avoid if the child has reflux or sensitivity to mint.

9. Quercetin (Natural Antihistamine, Age 4+)

Rationale:

Quercetin is a plant-based compound that reduces histamine release and inflammation, supporting the body's natural response to allergens and congestion.

Instructions:

a. Choose a pediatric-specific quercetin supplement or blend (such as D-Hist Jr.).
b. Follow dosing instructions or provider recommendations.
c. Offer with food for best absorption.

Precaution:

- May cause mild digestive upset or headaches.
- Introduce one supplement at a time to monitor tolerance.

10. Saline Nasal Irrigation

Rationale:

Saline rinses clear nasal passages of allergens, mucus, and irritants, supporting sinus health and moisture balance.

Instructions:

a. Use a sterile saline spray or nasal irrigation system.
b. For older children, a bulb syringe or spray bottle may be used.
c. Repeat 1–2 times daily or after outdoor exposure.

Precaution:

- Always use distilled, sterile, or boiled and cooled water.
- Not appropriate for infants without provider approval.

11. Steam Inhalation Therapy

Rationale:

Steam loosens thick mucus, reduces inflammation, and opens the sinuses. It can be enhanced with essential oils for further decongestant effects.

Instructions:

a. Add 3–5 drops of child-safe essential oil to a bowl of boiled water.
b. Have the child inhale the steam with a towel over their head for 5–10 minutes.
c. Alternatively, sit in a steamy bathroom with the shower running.

Precaution:

- Never leave a child unattended near hot water.
- Ensure essential oils used are safe for children and diluted properly.

12. Warm Chest Compress

Rationale:

Warmth promotes circulation and can help relax chest and sinus tension that often accompany nasal congestion.

Instructions:

a. Apply a clean, warm, damp cloth to the chest for 10 minutes.
b. Repeat as needed, particularly before bedtime.

Precaution:

- Always test the compress to ensure it's not too hot.
- Avoid if the child has a fever or skin irritation in the area.

13. Warm Foot Soak with Epsom Salt

Rationale:

Warming the feet can help redirect circulation and support sinus drainage via reflexive pathways in the body.

Instructions:

a. Fill a basin with warm water and add 1 tablespoon of Epsom salt.
b. Soak feet for 10–15 minutes before bed.
c. Optional: Add 1 drop lavender essential oil for calming effects (age 3+).

Precaution:

- Supervise to prevent slipping.
- Do not use if child has open cuts or foot irritation.

Nose Bleeds (Epistaxis)

A nosebleed (epistaxis) is the loss of blood from the tissues inside the nose caused by the rupture of small blood vessels in the nasal lining.

Causes:

- Dry Air (Indoor heating and low humidity)
- Nose Picking
- Frequent nose blowing
- Colds, Allergies & Sinus Infections
- Nasal Injuries (falls, bumps, or trauma)
- Foreign Objects
- Medications (overuse of nasal sprays)
- Rarely do medical conditions, such as blood clotting disorders, occur.

Signs & Symptoms:

- Bleeding from one or both nostrils
- Sensation of liquid flowing down the throat

Seek Immediate Medical Attention:

- The child loses a lot of blood or appears weak/dizzy.
- Frequent nosebleeds without a clear cause.
- Bleeding occurs after a head injury.
- Nose bleeds lasting more than 15-20 minutes, despite applying pressure.

How to Stop a Nosebleed:

Stay Calm & Comfort the Child – Reassure them that nosebleeds are common and not dangerous.

1. ***Positioning***
    a. Have the child **sit upright** (not lie down) to prevent swallowing blood.
    b. **Lean slightly forward** to avoid blood going down the throat.

2. ***Pinch the Nose***
    a. Using your thumb and index finger, pinch the soft part of the nose (just below the bony bridge).
    b. Keep firm pressure for 5-10 minutes without releasing.

3. ***Apply Cold Compress:***
    a. Place a cold pack or ice wrapped in a cloth on the bridge of the nose to help constrict blood vessels.

4. ***Encourage Breathing Through the Mouth – Avoid sniffing or blowing the nose for several hours.***
5. ***Moisturize the Nasal Passages:***
    a. Use a saline spray or apply petroleum jelly inside the nostrils if the air is dry.

6. ***Prevent Future Nosebleeds:***
    a. Keep the child's nails trimmed to avoid nose-picking.
    b. Use a humidifier in dry environments.
    c. Teach them to avoid blowing their nose too hard.

7. ***Cayenne Pepper Remedy (Do not do this with young children).***
    a. Mix **a pinch of cayenne pepper** in **warm water** and drink it.

Foreign Objects in the Nose

Safe Removal Tips:

1. Have the child **breathe through their mouth** to avoid inhaling further.
2. Try the **"Parent's Kiss" Method:**
   - Close the unaffected nostril.
   - Take a deep breath, **seal your lips around your child's mouth**, and give a firm puff of air.

If you cannot safely remove the object, take the child to urgent care or the emergency room for removal.

Allergies (Seasonal & Environmental)

Childhood allergies are immune hypersensitivity reactions to harmless substances such as pollen, dust mites, mold spores, or pet dander. In sensitive children, these allergens trigger the release of histamine and other inflammatory chemicals, leading to symptoms that affect the respiratory system, skin, and eyes. While antihistamines are commonly used, many families benefit from natural approaches that support immune regulation and reduce allergic responses.

Causes of Allergies:

- Seasonal pollen from trees, grasses, and weeds
- Indoor allergens such as dust mites, mold, and pet dander
- Environmental irritants (e.g., smoke, strong fragrances, pollution)
- Food sensitivities (especially dairy, eggs, peanuts)
- Weather or climate shifts (cold fronts, humidity, barometric pressure)

Signs and Symptoms of Allergies:

In Infants & Toddlers:

- Nasal congestion or sneezing
- Runny nose with clear discharge
- Red, watery, or itchy eyes
- Skin rashes or eczema flare-ups
- Fussiness or disrupted sleep

In Older Children:

- Frequent sneezing or postnasal drip
- Itchy eyes, ears, throat, or nose
- Nasal congestion or sinus pressure
- Headaches or persistent fatigue
- Difficulty concentrating in school

- Dry cough, mild wheezing, or throat clearing

When to Seek Medical Attention:

Seek prompt evaluation if any of the following occur:

- Symptoms last longer than 2–3 weeks without improvement
- Difficulty breathing, chest tightness, or wheezing
- Swelling of the face or lips, widespread hives, or signs of anaphylaxis
- Ongoing sleep disturbances due to cough or congestion
- Behavioral changes, poor appetite, or signs of discomfort
- No improvement with natural or over-the-counter treatments

Allergies vs. Asthma: Know the Difference

Allergies primarily affect the upper respiratory tract and skin, while asthma involves inflammation of the lower airways. If your child experiences persistent coughing, chest tightness, or wheezing, particularly at night or early in the morning, these may be signs of asthma rather than allergies. Unlike typical allergy symptoms, asthma can disrupt sleep and impair breathing. A medical evaluation is essential to confirm the diagnosis and initiate appropriate treatment, especially if nighttime symptoms or exercise intolerance are present.

Note: Do not give honey to children under 1 year old due to the risk of botulism.

Why Local Raw Honey is Best for Allergies:

When dealing with seasonal allergies, using local raw honey is one of the most effective natural remedies. Local honey works because it contains trace amounts of local pollen. When consumed regularly, this pollen acts as a "natural vaccine," gradually helping your body build tolerance to the allergens in your environment.

Rationale:

- Local honey contains small amounts of pollen from flowers and plants in your region.
- When consumed in small, consistent amounts, it introduces these allergens to your immune system in a mild form.
- Over time, your body builds immunity to these allergens, reducing seasonal allergy symptoms such as sneezing, congestion, and watery eyes.
- For best results, take ½ to 1 teaspoon of local raw honey daily, starting a few months before allergy season.

Not All Honey is Created Equal – Avoid Fake Honey!

Many store-bought honey brands are highly processed and contain little to no real honey. Some brands mix cheap fillers like high-fructose corn syrup, which unnecessarily removes honey's natural health benefits and even spikes blood sugar levels.

How to Spot Fake Honey:

- If the label lists "high-fructose corn syrup" or "glucose syrup," it's not pure honey.
- Ultra-filtered honey (clear, without pollen particles) is often stripped of nutrients.
- Real honey does not dissolve immediately in water; it sinks before dissolving.
- Pure honey thickens or crystallizes over time—if your honey never thickens, it may be diluted.

Buy raw, unfiltered honey from a trusted source, preferably a local beekeeper or farmers' market.

Natural Remedies for Pediatric Allergies

1. Butterbur (Petasites hybridus)

Rationale:

Butterbur is a botanical extract with antihistamine and leukotriene-blocking effects. It has been shown in clinical studies to reduce nasal congestion, sneezing, and other allergic symptoms.

Instructions:

a. Use only PA-free (pyrrolizidine alkaloid-free) standardized formulations approved for pediatric use.
b. Consult a qualified healthcare provider before use to ensure age-appropriate dosing and safety.

Precaution:

- Do not use raw or unprocessed butterbur due to the risk of liver toxicity.
- Only administer PA-free formulations labeled for children under professional guidance.

2. D-Hist Jr.

Rationale:

This pediatric chewable supplement contains quercetin, stinging nettle, bromelain, vitamin C, and N-acetylcysteine (NAC). It supports mast cell stabilization, modulates histamine release, and promotes upper respiratory health. Quercetin and stinging nettle act as natural antihistamines, while bromelain and NAC aid in mucus thinning and inflammation reduction.

Instructions:

a. Administer 1–2 chewables daily with food, following age-appropriate dosing on the product label.

Precaution:

- Ensure the child is able to safely chew the tablet.
- Monitor for signs of allergy or gastrointestinal discomfort when first introduced.

3. HEPA Air Purifiers

Rationale:

HEPA filtration captures microscopic particles, including pollen, pet dander, and dust mites, improving air quality and reducing allergen load.

Instructions:

a. Place air purifiers in the child's bedroom and main living spaces.
b. Use continuously during high-allergen seasons and replace filters as directed.

Precaution:

- Avoid air purifiers that generate ozone or use ionizers, as these may irritate sensitive lungs in children.

4. Local Bee Pollen (for children over 2 years)

Rationale:

Bee pollen introduces small amounts of local allergens to the immune system, helping to promote tolerance and reduce sensitivity to environmental triggers.

Instructions:

a. Start with a few granules under the tongue and slowly increase to ¼–½ teaspoon daily.
b. Ensure the pollen is raw and locally sourced.

Precaution:

- Introduce slowly and monitor for signs of allergic reaction (rash, swelling, or breathing difficulty).
- Discontinue immediately if any reaction occurs.

5. *Local Raw Honey (1+)*

Rationale:

Local raw honey contains trace pollen that may gradually reduce the immune system's overreaction to allergens. It mimics natural desensitization similar to immunotherapy.

Instructions:

a. Give ½ to 1 teaspoon daily, ideally year-round.
b. Ensure the honey is raw, unfiltered, and sourced locally.

Precaution:

- Do not give to children under 12 months due to risk of botulism.
- Always supervise ingestion to prevent choking in toddlers.

6. *Nettle Tea (Age 3+)*

Rationale:

Stinging nettle is a natural antihistamine and anti-inflammatory herb traditionally used to ease sneezing, nasal congestion, and itching related to allergies.

Instructions:

a. Steep 1 teaspoon of dried nettle leaf in 1 cup of hot water for 10 minutes, then strain.
b. Cool to a safe temperature before offering.
c. Offer small sips once daily during allergy season.

Precaution:

- Not recommended for children under 3.
- Introduce slowly and monitor for sensitivity or upset stomach.

7. Probiotics

Rationale:

Probiotics support gut health, which plays a critical role in immune system regulation and allergic response. They are especially beneficial in children with eczema or recent antibiotic use.

Instructions:

a. Select a refrigerated, high-quality pediatric formulation containing strains such as *Lactobacillus rhamnosus GG* or *Bifidobacterium infantis*.
b. Administer daily according to the label or pediatric recommendation.

Precaution:

- Choose only age-appropriate products.
- Some children may initially experience mild gas or bloating, which typically resolves with continued use.

8. Quercetin (Stand-alone or in Blends)

Rationale:

Quercetin is a bioflavonoid with anti-inflammatory and mast cell-stabilizing properties. It helps reduce histamine release and allergic symptoms when taken regularly.

Instructions:

a. Use only quercetin supplements labeled for pediatric use.
b. Follow provider-recommended dosing and observe for individual tolerance.

Precaution:

- May cause mild headaches or digestive upset in sensitive children.
- Introduce gradually and avoid combining with multiple new suppleBments at once.

9. Saline Nasal Rinse or Spray

Rationale:

Saline solutions flush allergens, pollen, and irritants from the nasal passages, reduce swelling, and support mucosal health.

Instructions:

a. Use a sterile saline spray, neti pot, or bulb syringe to rinse the nostrils.
b. Perform once or twice daily, especially after outdoor exposure.

Precaution:

- Use only distilled, sterile, or previously boiled and cooled water for rinses.
- Avoid using pressurized sprays in infants or very young children.

CHAPTER 03

MOUTH & THROAT

This section is for educational purposes only. The remedies listed are intended to support comfort and wellness and should not be used as a substitute for professional medical advice. Always consult your child's healthcare provider for diagnosis and treatment.

Sore Throat (Pharyngitis), Tonsillitis & Strep Throat

A **sore throat** is inflammation or irritation of the throat (pharynx), often caused by **viral infections**, but also triggered by **allergies**, **dry air**, or **irritants**. Viral sore throats typically resolve independently, but proper care and symptom relief can speed recovery and prevent discomfort.

Causes

- **Viral infections** (cold, flu, mononucleosis, COVID-19)
- **Bacterial infections** (Group A Streptococcus)
- **Allergies** (pollen, dust, pet dander)
- **Irritants** (smoke, pollution, dry air)
- **Acid reflux (GERD)**
- **Vocal strain** (yelling, excessive speaking)

Signs & Symptoms

In Infants & Toddlers:

- Irritability or increased crying
- Trouble swallowing or refusal to eat
- Excessive drooling
- Fever (more likely in bacterial cases)
- Swollen neck glands
- Foul breath

Older Children May Experience:

- **Throat pain, especially when swallowing**
- **Swollen, red tonsils**, possibly with white patches
- **Hoarseness** or **muffled voice**
- **Fatigue**, headache, body aches
- **Nausea or abdominal pain** (common with strep)

Seek Immediate Medical Attention:

- Fever exceeds **102°F (38.9°C)** or lasts longer than 3 days

- **Swallowing is difficult** or child is drooling
- White patches on tonsils or red rash on body
- **Swollen glands** or **neck stiffness**
- **Symptoms persist beyond 10–14 days**

Natural Remedies for Sore Throat (Pharyngitis)

1. Chamomile Tea (Age 6+ or under guidance)

Rationale:

Chamomile has anti-inflammatory and mild analgesic properties. It soothes irritated throat tissues, relaxes muscles, and may help reduce discomfort and promote rest during illness.

Instructions:

a. Steep 1 chamomile tea bag or 1 tsp dried chamomile flowers in 1 cup of hot water for 5–10 minutes.
b. Allow to cool to a safe drinking temperature.
c. Offer in small sips, up to 1–2 times daily during acute symptoms.

Precaution:

- Not recommended for children under 6 unless approved by a healthcare provider.
- Avoid if allergic to ragweed or related plants.

2. Cool Mist Humidifier

Rationale:

Moist air helps soothe a dry, irritated throat and supports respiratory comfort, especially during sleep or in heated indoor environments.

Instructions:

a. Place a cool mist humidifier near the child's bed or play area.
b. Run it during naps and overnight during illness.
c. Clean the device daily to prevent mold and bacterial growth.

Precaution:

- Use only distilled water to reduce mineral buildup.
- Avoid warm mist models to prevent burns in children.

3. *Licorice Root Tea (Age 5+)*

Rationale:

Licorice root has antiviral and demulcent properties that soothe and coat the throat lining. It may also reduce inflammation and ease coughing.

Instructions:

a. Steep 1 tsp dried licorice root in 1 cup hot water for 5–10 minutes.
b. Strain and allow to cool to a warm, safe temperature.
c. Offer ¼ to ½ cup once or twice daily during sore throat episodes.

Precaution:

- Not for prolonged use or in children under age 5.
- Avoid in children with high blood pressure, adrenal issues, or under medical treatment without provider guidance.

4. *Marshmallow Root Tea*

Rationale:

Marshmallow root contains mucilage, a gel-like substance that coats and protects inflamed throat tissues, reducing irritation and discomfort.

Instructions:

a. Add 1 tablespoon dried marshmallow root to 1 cup hot water.
b. Steep covered for 10–15 minutes.
c. Strain and cool to a warm temperature. Add honey for taste if desired.
d. Offer ¼ to ½ cup 2–3 times daily during symptoms.

Precaution:

- Ensure product is food-grade and clean.
- Always supervise when serving herbal teas to younger children.

5. Oregano Oil (Age 5+)

Rationale:

Oregano oil contains carvacrol and thymol, natural compounds with strong antimicrobial, antiviral, and anti-inflammatory effects, helpful during infection.

Instructions:

a. Dilute 1–2 drops oregano oil in 1 teaspoon olive oil or raw honey.
b. Give once daily for up to 5 days.
c. Administer at mealtime to minimize strong taste and digestive upset.

Precaution:

- Never give undiluted oregano oil.
- Not for children under age 5 unless specifically approved by a healthcare provider.
- Monitor for gastrointestinal upset or sensitivity.

6. *Saltwater Gargle (Age 4+)*

Rationale:

Saltwater helps reduce swelling, draw out irritants, and gently disinfect the throat lining. It also loosens mucus and promotes healing.

Instructions:

a. Mix 1 teaspoon of quality salt (Himalayan, Celtic, or sea salt) in 8 ounces of warm water.
b. Have the child gargle and spit out without swallowing.
c. Repeat up to 3 times daily, especially after meals.

Precaution:

- Only suitable for children old enough to gargle safely.
- Always supervise to avoid accidental swallowing.

7. *Slippery Elm Lozenges (Age 4+)*

Rationale:

Slippery elm contains mucilage that forms a soothing film over sore or inflamed throat tissues, reducing irritation and pain.

Instructions:

a. Use lozenges or tablets specifically labeled for children.
b. Allow child to slowly dissolve in the mouth up to 3 times daily during sore throat episodes.

Precaution:

- Do not give to children under age 4 due to choking risk.
- Avoid if child has tree pollen allergies or known sensitivity to elm.

8. Warm Honey-Lemon Water (Age 1+)

Rationale:

Honey has antimicrobial properties and soothes throat tissues, while lemon provides vitamin C and helps break up mucus.

Instructions:

a. Mix 1 teaspoon of raw honey with the juice of ¼ lemon in 1 cup of warm water.
b. Stir well and allow child to sip slowly.
c. Offer 2–3 times daily during acute symptoms.

Precaution:

- Never give honey to children under 12 months due to the risk of infant botulism.
- Ensure water is warm, not hot.

Tonsillitis

Tonsillitis is inflammation of the tonsils, often caused by the same viruses that cause colds or bacterial infections like strep. Symptoms include **throat pain**, **swollen tonsils**, and **difficulty swallowing**.

Causes

- **Viruses** (adenovirus, influenza, RSV)
- **Bacterial**: Group A Streptococcus

Signs & Symptoms

a. Swollen, red, or pus-covered tonsils
b. **Painful swallowing**
c. **Fever and bad breath**
d. **Neck lymph node swelling**
e. Snoring or trouble sleeping (in severe cases)

When to Seek Medical Attention

- High fever with white patches on the tonsils
- Difficulty swallowing or speaking
- **Recurrent tonsillitis** (6+ times/year)
- Breathing or sleep disturbances due to swollen tonsils

Natural Remedies for Tonsillitis

1. *Cold Treats*

Rationale:

Cold reduces blood flow to inflamed tissues, helping to numb pain and reduce swelling. It provides fast, temporary relief for acute throat discomfort.

Instructions:

a. Offer cold foods such as popsicles, frozen fruit, or small ice chips (age-appropriate).
b. Allow the child to suck slowly for maximum soothing effect.
c. Use several times a day during periods of acute throat pain.

Precaution:

- Always supervise young children with ice or frozen treats to prevent choking.
- Avoid overly sugary popsicles or those with artificial dyes, which may worsen inflammation.

2. Turmeric Milk (Age 2+)

Rationale:

Turmeric contains curcumin, which offers natural anti-inflammatory, antimicrobial, and immune-supportive properties. When mixed with warm milk, it also soothes the throat lining and promotes rest.

Instructions:

a. Warm 1 cup of milk on the stove or in a safe container (do not boil).
b. Stir in ½ teaspoon of turmeric powder.
c. Optional: Add ½ teaspoon of raw honey if the child is over 1 year old.
d. Serve once daily, preferably before bedtime.

Precaution:

- Not for use in children with turmeric allergies or dairy intolerance.
- Ensure milk is warm, not hot, to avoid burns.

3. Licorice Root Tea (Age 5+)

Rationale:

Licorice root acts as a demulcent, forming a soothing coating over sore throat tissues. It also has mild antiviral and anti-inflammatory properties, which may help relieve pain and irritation.

Instructions:

a. Steep 1 teaspoon of dried licorice root in 1 cup of boiling water for 10 minutes.
b. Strain and cool to a safe, warm temperature.
c. Offer up to ½ cup twice daily during throat discomfort.

Precaution:

- Not recommended for long-term use or for children with high blood pressure.
- Always use in moderation and under supervision.

4. Oregano Oil (Age 5+)

See number 5 under sore throat (Pharyngitis) instructions above.

5. Saltwater Gargle (Age 4+)

See number 6 under sore throat (Pharyngitis) instructions above.

Strep Throat

Strep throat is a bacterial infection caused by *Group A Streptococcus*. It requires **antibiotic treatment** to avoid serious complications and reduce contagiousness.

Causes

- *Group A Streptococcus* bacteria
- Spread through respiratory droplets or contact with contaminated surfaces

Signs & Symptoms

- Sudden onset sore throat
- Painful swallowing
- Fever above **101°F (38.3°C)**
- White or yellow patches on the tonsils
- Swollen, tender lymph nodes
- Absence of cough or nasal symptoms

How to Identify

Strep throat causes intense throat pain, fever, and white patches on the tonsils without cold symptoms. A rapid strep test is necessary to confirm the diagnosis.

Seek Immediate Medical Attention:

- High fever and sore throat without runny nose or cough
- Red rash or white coating on tongue (scarlet fever)
- Known exposure to strep throat
- The child is not eating, drinking, or speaking due to pain

Why Antibiotics Are Necessary

An untreated strep infection can lead to:

- **Rheumatic fever** (affects the heart and joints)
- **Kidney inflammation** (post-streptococcal glomerulonephritis)
- **Peritonsillar abscess** (serious tonsil complication)
- Ear or Sinus Infection

Antibiotics reduce symptom duration, prevent complications, and stop contagion within **24 hours** of beginning treatment.

Natural Remedies for Strep Throat (Supportive)

Natural remedies for strep throat focus on soothing sore throat pain, boosting the immune system, and reducing inflammation. These remedies can be used alongside antibiotics or as comfort care while awaiting diagnosis, but they should never delay medical treatment when strep is suspected.

1. Bone Broth

Rationale:

Bone broth provides essential minerals, collagen, and amino acids that support healing and comfort during illness. It also keeps the throat moist and nourished.

Instructions:

a. Warm homemade or high-quality bone broth to a safe drinking temperature.
b. Offer in small sips throughout the day.
c. Preparation instructions can be found in Chapter 11: Immune Support.

Precaution:

- Avoid bouillon cubes or commercial broths with added preservatives or MSG.

2. Elderberry Syrup

Rationale:

Elderberry is rich in antioxidants and flavonoids that support immune function. It may help reduce the severity and duration of viral illnesses and soothe throat inflammation.

Instructions:

a. Use a high-quality commercial or homemade elderberry syrup (see recipe in Chapter 11: Immune Support).
b. Give ½ to 1 teaspoon once or twice daily depending on the child's age and product instructions.

Precaution:

- Choose products with minimal added sugars.
- Do not exceed recommended dosage.

3. Ginger Tea (Age 2+)

Rationale:

Ginger is a natural anti-inflammatory and can ease throat pain, support immunity, and reduce nausea that may accompany illness.

Instructions:

a. Simmer several thin slices of fresh ginger root in 1 cup of water for 10 minutes.
b. Strain and sweeten with raw honey (if child is over 1 year).
c. Serve warm in small sips.

Precaution:

- Avoid if the child has a history of reflux or ginger sensitivity.
- Use mild strength to prevent strong, spicy taste.

4. *Marshmallow Root Tea (Age 1+)*

Rationale:

Marshmallow root is high in mucilage, which coats and soothes inflamed throat tissues, reducing pain and irritation.

Instructions:

a. Steep 1 teaspoon of dried marshmallow root in 1 cup of warm (not boiling) water for 10 minutes.
b. Strain and cool to a safe temperature.
c. Offer in small sips throughout the day.

Precaution:

- Always ensure tea is cool enough for safe drinking.
- Use food-grade herbs from trusted sources.

5. *Oregano Oil (Age 5+)*

Rationale:

See 5 under Sore Throat (Pharyngitis) for full instructions. Has natural antibacterial and immune-boosting properties.

6. *Probiotics*

Rationale:

Probiotics help maintain gut flora balance during illness, especially during or after antibiotics. They may also reduce inflammation and support overall immune health.

Instructions:

a. Choose a pediatric probiotic containing strains such as Lactobacillus rhamnosus GG or Bifidobacterium infantis.
b. Give once or twice daily, at least 2 hours apart from antibiotics.

Precaution:

- Introduce slowly to monitor tolerance.
- Some children may experience mild gas or bloating initially.

7. Rest and Humidified Air

Rationale:

Rest promotes recovery, while humidified air soothes dry throat and nasal passages, especially during sleep.

Instructions:

a. Encourage extra sleep and reduced stimulation during illness.
b. Run a clean cool-mist humidifier in the child's room, especially overnight.
c. Clean the humidifier daily to prevent mold and bacterial buildup.

Precaution:

- Do not use warm-mist humidifiers around young children due to burn risk.
- Always use distilled water to reduce mineral buildup in the device.

8. Salt Water Gargle (Age 4+)

Rationale:

See 6 under Sore Throat (Pharyngitis) for full instructions. Helps reduce swelling, flush bacteria, and ease throat pain.

9. Throat Spray (Propolis or Colloidal Silver-Based)

Rationale:

Propolis has natural antibacterial and anti-inflammatory properties. Colloidal silver may reduce bacterial load when used occasionally. Both can offer targeted pain relief.

Instructions:

a. Choose a high-quality child-safe throat spray containing propolis or colloidal silver.
b. Spray directly onto the back of the throat 2–3 times per day as needed.

Precaution:

- Do not use silver products long-term.
- Always choose well-sourced, tested products.
- Avoid use if the child dislikes sprays or has a strong gag reflex.

10. Warm Lemon Water with Manuka Honey (Age 1+)

Rationale:

Lemon juice provides vitamin C and has natural astringent properties. Manuka honey coats and soothes the throat while offering potent antimicrobial effects.

Instructions:

a. Mix the juice of ½ lemon into 1 cup of warm (not hot) water.
b. Stir in 1 teaspoon of manuka honey.
c. Offer in small sips up to 2–3 times per day.

Precaution:

- Do not give honey to children under 12 months.
- Ensure water is warm—not hot—to avoid burns.

Seek Immediate Medical Attention

Strep throat, caused by *Group A Streptococcus*, can lead to serious complications, including rheumatic fever, kidney inflammation, and peritonsillar abscess. Unlike viral sore throats, strep requires antibiotics to prevent these risks, reduce symptoms, and stop the spread. If your child has a sore throat with fever, swollen glands, or white patches on the tonsils, they should be seen by a pediatrician or urgent care provider for a rapid strep test.

Oral Thrush & Mouth Sores

Oral thrush in infants is a yeast infection caused by *Candida albicans*. It can affect both the baby's mouth and the mother's nipples, creating a cycle of reinfection. It is common in breast-feeding infants.

You can gently check for **oral thrush in a baby at home** using the **"light scrape" method**, which helps distinguish thrush from milk residue. Here's how to do it **safely and effectively**:

How to Identify Oral Thrush Using the Light Scrape Method

What You'll Need:

- A clean, damp **washcloth** or **sterile cotton swab**
- Good lighting

Step-by-Step:

1. **Wash your hands thoroughly.**
2. **Look inside your baby's mouth:**
   - Check for **white patches** on the **tongue, inner cheeks, gums, or roof of the mouth**.
   - Thrush often looks like **creamy white or yellowish spots**, not just a coating.
3. **Gently rub one of the patches** with a damp washcloth or cotton swab.
4. **Observe the results**: If it's milk residue, it usually wipes away easily to reveal pink, healthy tissue and is typically limited to the tongue. In contrast, oral thrush is difficult to remove, may expose red or irritated tissue that can bleed, and often appears on the tongue, cheeks, lips, or gums.

Caution:

- **Never scrape hard**; you're not trying to remove the patch, test if it lifts easily.
- If your baby seems uncomfortable or has bleeding, **stop immediately**.

When to Suspect Thrush:

- Baby has **fussiness when feeding** or a poor latch.
- Patches return quickly after wiping
- You notice **diaper rash** or **yeast on your nipples.**

Natural Remedies for Oral Thrush

Oral thrush is a fungal infection caused by the overgrowth of *Candida albicans* in the mouth. It commonly affects infants, nursing mothers, and immunocompromised individuals. Natural remedies can offer safe, effective support in mild cases or alongside conventional treatments. Always consult a healthcare provider before beginning treatment in newborns.

1. Apple Cider Vinegar Rinse (For Older Children or Adults)

Rationale:

Apple cider vinegar has mild antifungal properties and helps rebalance the pH of the mouth, creating an environment less favorable for yeast overgrowth.

Instructions:

a. Mix 1 tablespoon of raw, unfiltered apple cider vinegar with ½ cup of water.
b. Swish the mixture in the mouth for 30 seconds to 1 minute, then spit it out.
c. Rinse the mouth with plain water afterward if desired.

Precaution:

- Not suitable for children under age 5 unless approved by a healthcare provider.
- Do not use more than 1–2 times daily.
- Discontinue use if burning or irritation occurs.

2. Coconut Oil Pulling (For Older Children or Nursing Mothers)

Rationale:

Coconut oil contains lauric acid, which has natural antifungal and antimicrobial properties. Oil pulling may help reduce oral fungal overgrowth and support oral hygiene in older children or mothers.

Instructions:

a. Swish 1 tablespoon of organic virgin coconut oil in the mouth for 5–10 minutes.
b. Spit the oil into the trash and rinse the mouth with warm water.
c. Perform once daily, ideally in the morning on an empty stomach.

Precaution:

- Not recommended for young children who may swallow the oil.
- Do not perform if there are oral motor difficulties or swallowing issues.
- Avoid spitting into drains, as coconut oil can solidify and cause clogs.

3. *Grapefruit Seed Extract (GSE) for Breastfeeding Mothers*

Rationale:

To prevent reinfection during infant oral thrush treatment, the mother's nipples should also be treated. Grapefruit seed extract has antifungal properties and helps eliminate *Candida* on the skin.

Instructions:

a. Dilute 5 drops of grapefruit seed extract in 1 ounce (30 mL) of distilled water.
b. After breastfeeding, apply the solution to each nipple and areola using a clean cotton pad or gauze.
c. Allow the area to air dry completely before covering with clothing or nursing again.
d. Optionally, rinse with warm water before the next feeding.
e. Apply 3 to 4 times daily until symptoms resolve and continue for a few days afterward to prevent recurrence.

Precaution:

- Ensure the area is fully dry before reapplying clothing.
- Discontinue use if cracking, burning, or irritation develops.

4. *Grapefruit Seed Extract (GSE) for Infants*

Rationale:

Grapefruit seed extract (GSE) contains bioflavonoids and polyphenols with antifungal and antimicrobial effects. When properly diluted, it can safely inhibit *Candida* growth in the mouth of infants.

Instructions:

a. Dilute 1 drop of grapefruit seed extract in 1 ounce (30 mL) of distilled water.

b. Use a clean cotton swab or finger cot to gently apply the solution to the tongue, gums, and inner cheeks.
c. Apply 2 to 3 times daily, ideally after feedings.
d. Alternatively, pour the diluted solution into a clean spray bottle and spray directly into the mouth if tolerated.

Precaution:

- Never use grapefruit seed extract undiluted.
- Test a small area for sensitivity before use.
- Discontinue if redness, fussiness, or irritation occurs.
- Not recommended in infants under 6 weeks without health-care provider guidance.

Teething

Teething is a natural developmental process during which an infant's primary teeth begin to erupt through the gums, typically starting between **4 to 7 months** of age. While it is a normal phase, teething can cause significant discomfort due to gum inflammation and pressure. Symptoms may vary from child to child and can occasionally mimic minor illnesses.

Signs & Symptoms of Teething

- Excessive drooling
- Swollen, tender, or red gums
- Desire to chew or gnaw on objects
- Fussiness or irritability
- Mild decrease in appetite
- Disrupted sleep or increased night waking
- Rubbing cheeks or pulling ears

When to Seek Medical Attention

- Fever above **100.4°F (38°C)** (not typical of teething alone)
- Diarrhea or persistent vomiting
- Refusal to eat or drink for prolonged periods
- Rash that spreads beyond the mouth or chin
- Signs of ear infection or illness unrelated to teething

Natural Remedies and Comfort Measures for Teething

1. *Amber Teething Necklaces*

Rationale:

Baltic amber is believed to release trace amounts of succinic acid when warmed by body heat. Some proponents suggest this may reduce inflammation and teething discomfort when worn close to the skin.

Instructions:

a. Use a child-sized amber necklace with a breakaway clasp.
b. Ensure it fits snugly but not tightly, and that it cannot be pulled into the mouth.
c. Supervise the child while wearing and remove during naps or sleep.

Precaution:

- Never allow the child to sleep with the necklace on.
- Do not allow chewing or pulling on the necklace.
- Ensure the necklace has a breakaway clasp to reduce strangulation risk.
- Always supervise while worn.

2. Breastfeeding (On Demand)

Rationale:

Breastfeeding provides comfort and pain relief through natural sucking and skin-to-skin contact. Nursing during teething helps reduce discomfort and may calm inflammation.

Instructions:

a. Offer the breast more frequently during teething flare-ups.
b. Allow for longer feeding sessions if the infant appears soothed.
c. Alternate nursing positions to ease gum pressure.

Precaution:

- Watch for signs of biting.
- Use cold compresses or nipple balm if the mother experiences irritation.

3. Chamomile Tea Compress or Teether Dip (Age 6 months+)

Rationale:

Chamomile is a natural anti-inflammatory and mild sedative that helps calm gum irritation and fussiness.

Instructions:

a. Steep 1 chamomile tea bag in hot water and allow it to cool completely.
b. Soak a clean washcloth in the tea or dip a clean teething toy into it.
c. Allow the baby to suck or chew under supervision.

Precaution:

- Use only in babies over 6 months.
- Ensure tea is organic and free from additives.
- Always supervise use.

4. Chilled Silicone Teething Rings or Toys

Rationale:

Cold pressure soothes inflamed gums and provides counter-stimulation to distract from discomfort.

Instructions:

a. Chill BPA-free or medical-grade silicone teething toys in the refrigerator.
b. Offer to the baby during teething episodes under supervision.
c. Wash and sanitize toys between each use.

Precaution:

- Avoid liquid- or gel-filled toys that may leak.
- Replace any toy that shows wear, cracks, or damage.
- Always supervise during use.

5. *Clean, Cold Washcloth*

Rationale:

A chilled, damp washcloth offers soft-textured pressure to inflamed gums while also providing cooling relief.

Instructions:

a. Moisten a clean washcloth with sterile or filtered water.
b. Chill in the refrigerator for 20–30 minutes.
c. Allow the baby to chew under supervision.

Precaution:

- Replace with a fresh cloth regularly to prevent bacterial growth.
- Always supervise to avoid gagging or choking.

6. *Clove Oil Gel (Age 2+)*

Rationale:

Clove oil contains eugenol, a natural compound with numbing and antimicrobial properties that can temporarily relieve gum pain when diluted.

Instructions:

a. Mix 1 drop of clove essential oil with 1 tablespoon of carrier oil (e.g., coconut oil).
b. Dip a clean fingertip or cotton swab into the mixture and apply gently to the gums.
c. Use no more than 1–2 times daily.

Precaution:

- For children over age 2 only.
- Must be extremely diluted.
- Discontinue if irritation, burning, or allergic reaction occurs.

7. Cold Chamomile Tea in Bottle or Sippy Cup (Age 6 months+)

Rationale:

Chilled chamomile tea offers gentle anti-inflammatory and calming support while hydrating and soothing sore gums.

Instructions:

a. Brew chamomile tea and refrigerate until cold.
b. Offer small sips in a bottle or sippy cup, particularly before naps.
c. Use alongside breast milk or formula, not as a replacement.

Precaution:

- Only for babies over 6 months.
- Ensure the tea is unsweetened and free from additives.
- Discard unused portions after a few hours.

8. Frozen Banana Chunks or Fruit in Mesh Feeder (Age 6 months+)

Rationale:

Cold fruit soothes swollen gums and encourages self-feeding. Mesh feeders minimize choking risk.

Instructions:

a. Cut a banana or soft fruit into small chunks and freeze.
b. Place frozen fruit into a mesh feeder and offer under supervision.
c. Clean the feeder thoroughly after use.

Precaution:

- Use only soft fruits.
- Check feeder for wear or damage.
- Discard uneaten fruit after each use.

9. Frozen Breast Milk Popsicles (Infants)

Rationale:

Breast milk provides immune-boosting, anti-inflammatory support. Frozen in popsicle form, it offers physical relief for sore gums.

Instructions:

a. Pour expressed breast milk into food-grade silicone pacifier molds or trays.
b. Freeze until solid and offer for sucking 2–3 times per day.
c. Always supervise use of frozen items.

Precaution:

- Use clean, sterile molds.
- Never leave the infant unattended.
- Discontinue if the infant struggles with cold sensitivity.

10. Gum Massage with Clean Finger

Rationale:

Gentle gum pressure increases circulation and eases teething discomfort naturally.

Instructions:

a. Wash hands thoroughly.
b. Use a clean finger or silicone fingertip brush to rub the baby's gums in slow, circular motions for 1–2 minutes.

Precaution:

- Avoid if gums appear broken, bleeding, or infected.
- Keep nails trimmed and fingers clean to prevent injury.

11. Licorice Root Stick (Age 1+)

Rationale:

Raw, unsweetened licorice root is firm and fibrous, offering a natural teething aid that can be chewed on safely under supervision.

Instructions:

a. Choose organic, whole licorice root sticks (not candy).
b. Offer one stick for chewing for 10–15 minutes at a time.
c. Supervise closely during use.

Precaution:

- Only use under adult supervision.
- Avoid in children with high blood pressure or certain health conditions.
- Discontinue if irritation or allergic reaction occurs.

Safety Reminder:

Always supervise infants during any teething intervention involving cold items, liquids, or small parts. Never freeze teething toys solid, and do not use topical numbing gels or medications unless prescribed by a healthcare provider.

Geographic Tongue

Geographic tongue is a benign condition characterized by smooth, red patches on the surface of the tongue bordered by white or light-colored edges. These patches can shift location over time and may cause sensitivity to spicy, acidic, or hot foods. Though harmless, geographic tongue may cause discomfort, especially in children.

Causes

- Genetic predisposition
- Emotional stress or illness
- Hormonal fluctuations
- Vitamin or mineral deficiencies (e.g., B12, zinc)
- Spicy or acidic foods
- Allergic or autoimmune triggers

Signs & Symptoms

- Irregular red patches on the surface of the tongue
- Sensitivity to certain foods
- Mild burning or irritation
- White or light borders around patches
- Shifting appearance over days or weeks

Seek Immediate Medical Attention:

- Tongue swelling or severe pain
- Pus, bleeding, or signs of infection
- Symptoms interfering with eating or drinking
- Lesions lasting longer than 10–14 days without improvement

Natural Remedies for Geographic Tongue

1. Aloe Vera Rinse

Rationale:

Aloe vera contains anti-inflammatory compounds and mucilage that coat and soothe irritated oral tissues. It can ease discomfort and promote healing of the tongue's surface.

Instructions:

a. Mix 1 teaspoon of food-grade aloe vera gel into ¼ cup of lukewarm water.
b. Have the child swish the solution gently in the mouth for 30 seconds, then spit it out.
c. Repeat 2–3 times daily, especially after meals or when discomfort is present.
d. Do not swallow unless the aloe product is clearly labeled as food-grade and safe for internal use.

Precaution:

- Use only aloe vera products labeled safe for oral or food use.
- Discontinue use if irritation worsens or develops.

2. Coconut Oil Pulling (Age 4+)

Rationale:

Coconut oil contains lauric acid, a natural antimicrobial and anti-inflammatory compound. Swishing with coconut oil can help coat irritated tongue tissue, reduce inflammation, and support healing.

Instructions:

a. Place ½ to 1 teaspoon of organic virgin coconut oil in the child's mouth.

b. Swish gently for 1–3 minutes (use shorter duration for younger children), then spit out and rinse with warm water.
c. Perform once daily, ideally in the morning before meals.

Precaution:

- Only for children age 4 and older who can swish and spit safely.
- Do not allow swallowing of the oil.
- Spit into a trash can, not the sink, to prevent plumbing issues.

3. Probiotics

Rationale:

Probiotics support the oral and gut microbiome, helping regulate immune responses and reduce inflammatory triggers that may contribute to geographic tongue flare-ups.

Instructions:

a. Choose pediatric probiotic lozenges, powders, or liquids containing strains such as *Lactobacillus rhamnosus* or *Bifidobacterium infantis*.
b. Follow the age-appropriate dosage on the label or as directed by a healthcare provider.
c. For younger children, mix probiotic powder into soft foods such as yogurt or milk.
d. Use once daily to support microbial balance.

Precaution:

- Introduce probiotics gradually to monitor for digestive changes.
- Consult a pediatric provider before use if the child is immunocompromised.

Additional Note:

When selecting probiotics, it is essential to choose products that are kept refrigerated during storage and shipping. High-quality probiotics often contain live, active cultures that are sensitive to heat. Exposure to elevated temperatures can significantly reduce their potency and effectiveness. To ensure maximum viability, look for probiotics labeled as "refrigerated" or shipped with cold packs to maintain a stable, cool temperature throughout transit.

Cold Sores in Children (Pediatric HSV-1)

Cold sores in children are caused by the **Herpes Simplex Virus Type 1 (HSV-1)**. These fluid-filled blisters typically appear **on or around the lips** and are contagious. Outbreaks may be triggered by **stress, fever, sun exposure, or immune suppression**. While antiviral medication may be prescribed for severe cases, many supportive and natural remedies can help relieve discomfort and promote healing in otherwise healthy children.

Signs & Symptoms of Cold Sores in Children

- Tingling, itching, or burning around the mouth (may be the first sign)
- Fluid-filled blisters or clusters of sores, often near the lips or chin
- Crusting over of sores within a few days
- Soreness or mild fever
- Swollen lymph nodes (occasionally)

When to Seek Medical Attention

- Sores persist longer than 10–14 days
- Difficulty eating, drinking, or speaking
- Child appears very ill or has a high fever
- Cold sores spread near or into the eyes
- Frequent recurrences if a child is immunocompromised

Natural Remedies for Cold Sores in Children

1. Aloe Vera Gel (All Ages)

Rationale:

Aloe vera provides gentle anti-inflammatory and antiviral effects. It cools irritated skin and supports healing of cold sore lesions.

Instructions:

a. Use pure, food-grade aloe vera gel with no added alcohol, dyes, or fragrance.
b. Apply a thin layer directly to the cold sore up to 4 times daily.
c. Safe for infants, toddlers, and older children.

Precaution:

- Perform a patch test before first use.
- Discontinue if redness, itching, or rash develops.

2. Cold Compress

Rationale:

Cold application reduces swelling, redness, and discomfort, especially during the early (tingling or itching) stage of a cold sore.

Instructions:

a. Soak a clean, soft cloth in cold water or chill it in the refrigerator.
b. Apply to the affected area for 10–15 minutes.
c. Repeat 3–4 times daily as needed for relief.

Precaution:

- Never apply ice directly to the skin.
- Always use a clean cloth to prevent contamination.

3. Frozen Breast Milk Popsicles (Infants & Toddlers)

Rationale:

Breast milk contains antibodies, antiviral compounds, and soothing factors. When frozen, it offers both immune support and cooling relief for infants experiencing oral cold sore discomfort.

Instructions:

a. Pour fresh expressed breast milk into a clean silicone pacifier or popsicle mold and freeze.
b. Offer for gentle sucking 2–3 times per day during symptoms.
c. Especially helpful during the early tingling or painful stage.

Precaution:

- Always supervise to prevent choking.
- Use only properly stored breast milk.

Canker Sores (Aphthous Ulcers)

Canker sores are small, shallow ulcers that develop inside the mouth, including the inner cheeks, lips, tongue, or gums. They are not contagious, and although the exact cause is unknown, common triggers include stress, mouth injury, food sensitivities, vitamin deficiencies, or immune reactions. Most resolve on their own in 7–10 days, but natural remedies can help reduce pain and speed healing.

Natural Remedies for Canker Sores

1. *Aloe Vera Gel (All Ages)*

Rationale:

Aloe vera contains anti-inflammatory and wound-healing compounds that help soothe oral irritation and support tissue regeneration.

Instructions:

a. Use food-grade, alcohol-free aloe vera gel.
b. Apply a small amount directly to the canker sore using a clean fingertip or swab.
c. Reapply 3–4 times daily, particularly after meals.

Precaution:

- Ensure the aloe product is labeled safe for oral use.
- Discontinue use if irritation increases.

2. *Baking Soda Paste*

Rationale:

Baking soda neutralizes acids in the mouth and may help dry out the sore, reducing discomfort and promoting healing.

Instructions:

a. Mix 1 teaspoon of baking soda with a few drops of water to form a thick paste.
b. Apply directly to the sore using a clean finger or cotton swab.
c. Leave on for 1–2 minutes, then rinse gently with water.
d. Use once or twice daily as needed.

Precaution:

- Discontinue if the child experiences burning or discomfort.
- Not recommended for use on bleeding or open sores.

3. Chamomile Tea Compress

Rationale:

Chamomile offers soothing and anti-inflammatory properties that can calm irritated tissue and support healing.

Instructions:

a. Steep 1 chamomile tea bag or 1 teaspoon dried chamomile flowers in hot water for 5 minutes.
b. Let the tea cool to a safe, warm temperature.
c. Soak a clean cotton swab or ball in the tea and apply to the sore for 1–2 minutes.
d. Repeat 2–3 times daily as needed.

Precaution:

- Always test the tea temperature before applying to avoid burns.
- Use organic, food-grade chamomile when possible.

4. Cold Compress or Ice Chips

Rationale:

Cold helps numb localized pain and reduce swelling or inflammation.

Instructions:

a. Apply a cold item such as an ice chip, frozen spoon, or breast milk pop directly to the sore for short intervals.
b. Repeat throughout the day as needed for relief.
c. Use only under adult supervision.

Precaution:

- Supervise young children to prevent choking.
- Avoid prolonged or direct application of ice.

5. *Coconut Oil (All Ages)*

Rationale:

Coconut oil contains lauric acid, known for its antimicrobial and soothing properties, making it helpful in promoting comfort and healing.

Instructions:

a. Dab a small amount of organic virgin coconut oil directly onto the sore with a clean swab.
b. Reapply 2–3 times daily.
c. Older children may swish a small amount and spit it out under supervision.

Precaution:

- Ensure oil is fresh and food-grade.
- Prevent young children from swallowing the oil.

6. *Honey Dab (Age 1+)*

Rationale:

Raw honey has antimicrobial and healing effects and can coat the sore, easing pain and irritation.

Instructions:

a. Use high-quality raw honey such as manuka or local, unfiltered varieties.
b. Dab a small amount directly onto the sore with a clean finger or swab.
c. Reapply 3–4 times daily, especially after meals or before bed.

Precaution:

- Do not use honey in children under 12 months due to botulism risk.

7. Nutritional Support (As Advised by Provider)

Rationale:

Recurrent or slow-healing canker sores may be linked to nutrient deficiencies. Addressing these imbalances can improve healing and reduce recurrence.

Instructions:

a. Provide a balanced diet rich in iron, folate, vitamin B12, and zinc.
b. Discuss supplementation with a pediatric provider if sores are frequent.
c. Maintain hydration and good oral hygiene during outbreaks.

Precaution:

- Only supplement under medical guidance, especially with iron or zinc.
- Monitor for improvement and consult if symptoms persist.

8. Saltwater Rinse (Age 3+)

Rationale:

Saltwater helps cleanse the mouth, reduce bacteria, and promote healing of irritated oral tissues.

Instructions:

a. Mix 1 teaspoon of salt into 1 cup (8 oz) of warm water.
b. Have the child swish gently for 30 seconds and then spit out.
c. Repeat 2–3 times daily, especially after meals and before bed.

Precaution:

- Not suitable for children under 3 or those who cannot reliably spit.
- Do not swallow the rinse.

Hand, Foot, and Mouth Disease (HFMD)

Hand, Foot, and Mouth Disease is a **highly contagious viral illness** most commonly caused by the **Coxsackievirus A16** or **Enterovirus 71**. It typically affects children under age 5 but can occur at any age. The infection is usually mild and self-limiting, but can cause significant discomfort due to painful mouth sores, skin rashes, and fever.

Signs & Symptoms of HFMD

- Low-grade **fever** (often the first sign)
- **Sore throat** or refusal to eat
- **Painful mouth sores** (tongue, gums, inner cheeks)
- **Rash on hands, feet**, and sometimes buttocks or legs
- **Irritability, drooling, or fatigue**

When to Seek Medical Attention

- Inability to swallow or drink due to mouth pain
- Dehydration (dry lips, no tears, fewer wet diapers)
- High fever **>102°F (38.9°C)** lasting more than 3 days
- Sores that become infected (pus, swelling, foul odor)
- Symptoms lasting **longer than 10 days**

Natural Remedies for Hand, Foot, and Mouth Disease

1. *Calendula Salve or Balm (All Ages)*

Rationale:

Calendula has anti-inflammatory and skin-soothing properties that help calm irritation and support healing of HFMD rashes.

Instructions:

a. Apply a thin layer of calendula balm to clean, intact skin 2–3 times daily.

b. Use only on areas without open blisters or wounds.

Precaution:

- Perform a patch test before full use.
- Discontinue if irritation or rash worsens.

2. Chamomile or Calendula Mouth Rinse (Age 2+)

Rationale:

Chamomile and calendula are gentle herbs known for their anti-inflammatory and soothing effects on irritated mucosal tissue.

Instructions:

- Steep 1 teaspoon of dried chamomile or calendula in 1 cup of hot water for 10 minutes.
- Cool completely to room temperature.
- For older children, swish gently and spit out 2–3 times daily.

a. For younger children, dab onto sores using a clean cloth or cotton swab.

Precaution:

- Do not swallow the rinse.
- Discard unused rinse after 24 hours.

3. Cold, Soft Foods

Rationale:

Soft and cool foods reduce pain from mouth sores while maintaining calorie intake and hydration.

Instructions:

a. Offer foods like smoothies, chilled applesauce, yogurt, pureed fruits, and homemade popsicles.
b. Avoid spicy, salty, or acidic foods that may increase pain.

c. Encourage hydration through water, herbal teas, or coconut water.

Precaution:

- Avoid force-feeding. Allow smaller, more frequent meals as tolerated.

4. Coconut Oil Swab (All Ages)

Rationale:

Coconut oil is soothing and has antiviral, antifungal, and moisturizing effects, making it useful for both oral and lip care in HFMD.

Instructions:

a. Apply a small amount of organic, virgin coconut oil to affected oral areas or lips using a clean cotton swab
b. Reapply 2–3 times daily or as needed. c) Safe to use during breastfeeding.

Precaution:

- Always use clean tools for application.
- Avoid contaminating the oil container.

5. Cool Chamomile Cloth Compress (All Ages)

Rationale:

Chamomile's calming and anti-inflammatory properties help reduce fever and soothe skin irritation or discomfort.

Instructions:

a. Brew a strong cup of chamomile tea and let it cool completely.
b. Soak a soft cloth in the tea, wring it out, and apply to the forehead, neck, or back.

c. Refresh as needed for soothing effect, especially during rest or fever.

Precaution:

- Ensure the cloth is not too cold before applying.
- Avoid covering the child's mouth or nose.

6. Elderberry Syrup (Age 1+)

Rationale:

Elderberry supports the immune system and provides antiviral benefits that may help reduce the severity or duration of HFMD.

Instructions:

a. Administer a properly prepared elderberry syrup once or twice daily during illness.
b. Follow the dosing on the label or consult a pediatric provider.
c. Use only products made from cooked or processed elderberries.

Precaution:

- Do not give raw or unprocessed elderberries.
- Avoid use in children with berry allergies.
- Do not exceed recommended dosage.

7. Frozen Breast Milk Popsicles (Infants & Toddlers)

Rationale:

Breast milk offers antiviral and anti-inflammatory support while providing soothing relief and hydration when frozen into popsicles.

Instructions:

a. Freeze expressed breast milk in food-grade silicone pacifier or popsicle molds.
b. Offer for gentle sucking 2–3 times per day for 5–10 minutes.
c. Especially helpful during oral pain or refusal to eat.

Precaution:

- Always supervise use to prevent choking.
- Use only fresh or properly stored breast milk.

8. Hydration Support

Rationale:

Maintaining hydration is critical during HFMD, especially when oral sores make drinking uncomfortable.

Instructions:

a. Encourage frequent small sips of water, breast milk, herbal tea, or bone broth.
b. Offer homemade electrolyte drinks (water with lemon, honey if age 1+, and a pinch of salt).
c. Use oral rehydration solutions if needed during diarrhea or reduced intake.

Precaution:

- Monitor for signs of dehydration: dry lips, sunken eyes, low urine output.
- Seek medical care if fluid intake stops for more than 12 hours.

9. Oatmeal Baths for Skin Rash (All Ages)

Rationale:

Colloidal oatmeal reduces itching and irritation from HFMD rash and supports overall skin healing.

Instructions:

a. Add 1 cup of colloidal oatmeal to a warm (not hot) bath.
b. Allow the child to soak for 15–20 minutes.
c. Gently pat skin dry afterward—do not rub.

Precaution:

- Always supervise during bath time.
- Use a non-slip mat to prevent slipping.

CHAPTER 04

EYES & HEAD

This section is for educational purposes only. The remedies listed are intended to support comfort and wellness and should not be used as a substitute for professional medical advice. Always consult your child's healthcare provider for diagnosis and treatment.

Pink Eye (Conjunctivitis)

Conjunctivitis, commonly known as **pink eye**, is the inflammation of the thin transparent membrane (conjunctiva) that lines the white part of the eye and inner eyelid. It is a common condition in infants and children and can be caused by **viral infections**, **bacterial infections**, or **allergic reactions**. While most cases are mild and self-limiting, proper care helps relieve symptoms and prevent spread.

Causes

- Viral infections (adenovirus, enterovirus, associated with colds)
- Bacterial infections (*Staphylococcus*, *Streptococcus*, *Haemophilus influenzae*)
- Allergens (pollen, dust, pet dander)
- Chemical irritants (chlorine, smoke, soap, shampoo)

Signs & Symptoms of Conjunctivitis:

- Redness in the white part of the eye or inner eyelid
- Watery, itchy, or burning eyes
- Crusting of the eyelids or lashes, especially upon waking
- Yellow or green discharge (suggests bacterial cause)
- Excessive tearing (more common in viral or allergic cases)
- Sensitivity to light or mild swelling around the eyes
- It may affect one or both eyes

Seek Immediate Medical Attention

Medical evaluation is recommended if the child has thick yellow or green discharge, fever, or increasing redness and swelling. Immediate care is necessary if symptoms worsen after 24–48 hours of home treatment, if the child has vision changes, extreme light sensitivity, or if symptoms involve both eyes in an infant. Newborns or babies under 2 months old with any eye redness or discharge should be seen by a pediatrician promptly, as this may indicate a more serious infection.

Natural Remedies for Viral or Irritant Conjunctivitis

1. *Breast Milk Drops*

Rationale:

Fresh breast milk contains immune-supportive compounds such as secretory IgA and lactoferrin, which may soothe and help reduce inflammation in mild cases of eye irritation.

Instructions:

a. Express a few drops of fresh breast milk into a sterile container.
b. Using a clean dropper, place 1–2 drops into the affected eye.
c. Apply 2–3 times daily using only freshly expressed milk.

Precaution:

- Use immediately after expressing.
- Discontinue use if redness, swelling, or discharge worsens.

2. *Chamomile Tea Compress (Age 6 months+)*

Rationale:

Chamomile has mild anti-inflammatory and calming effects that can soothe irritation when used externally around the eye.

Instructions:

a. Steep 1 chamomile tea bag in 1 cup of hot water for 5 minutes.
b. Allow to cool completely, then soak a clean cloth in the tea.
c. Lay the cloth over the closed eye for 5–10 minutes.

d. Use a fresh tea bag or cloth for each eye and treatment.

Precaution:

- For external use only. Do not use chamomile tea as eye drops.
- Discontinue use if allergic symptoms (e.g., swelling, rash) occur.

3. *Cold Compress for Itching and Swelling*

Rationale:

Cold compresses help reduce puffiness, redness, and itchiness commonly seen with allergic or irritant conjunctivitis.

Instructions:

a. Soak a clean washcloth in cold water or chill a cloth in the refrigerator.
b. Gently place the compress over the closed eye for 5–10 minutes.
c. Repeat 2–3 times daily or as needed for relief.

Precaution:

- Never apply ice directly to the eye.
- Use a clean cloth for each eye to prevent cross-contamination.

4. *Immune Support (If Viral Conjunctivitis Suspected)*

Rationale:

If conjunctivitis is caused by a virus, supporting the immune system may help reduce duration and severity.

Instructions:

a. Offer foods rich in vitamin C (berries, bell peppers), zinc (legumes, seeds), and healthy fluids.

b. Encourage rest and reduce screen time to prevent additional eye strain.
c. Consider pediatric probiotics or multivitamins under provider guidance.

Precaution:

- Avoid supplements not formulated for children.
- Monitor for signs of bacterial superinfection (yellow discharge, increased pain, swelling).

5. Non-Tear Baby Wash Eye Rinse

Rationale:

A diluted tear-free baby shampoo solution may help clean the eyelid area and remove discharge, allergens, or irritants without stinging.

Instructions:

a. Mix 1 drop of tear-free baby wash into 1 cup of sterile, boiled, or distilled water.
b. Soak a clean cotton ball or pad in the solution.
c. Gently wipe from the inner corner to the outer edge of the affected eye.
d. Use a fresh cotton ball for each swipe and each eye.
e. Repeat 2–3 times daily as needed.

Precaution:

- Do not apply the solution directly into the eye.
- Discontinue use if irritation worsens.

6. Saline Eye Drops or Rinse

Rationale:

Sterile saline rinses help flush the eye and remove dust, allergens, or mucus. They provide gentle, non-medicated relief for viral or irritant conjunctivitis.

Instructions:

a. Use preservative-free, sterile saline eye drops.
b. Administer 1–2 drops into the affected eye every 4 hours as needed.
c. Discard the bottle 30 days after opening or if contaminated.

Precaution:

- Avoid touching the bottle tip to the eye or lashes.
- Use a separate bottle for each child if treating more than one.

7. Warm Compress

Rationale:

Warm compresses can soothe irritation, promote drainage, and help loosen crusty discharge common with viral or irritant conjunctivitis.

Instructions:

a. Soak a clean, soft cloth in warm (not hot) water and wring out excess moisture.
b. Gently place over the closed eye for 5–10 minutes.
c. Use a fresh cloth for each eye and each treatment.
d. Repeat 2–3 times daily or as needed for comfort.

Precaution:

- Do not reuse cloths between eyes or sessions.
- Check the temperature to ensure it's safe before applying.

Stye (Hordeolum)

A **stye** is a red, swollen, and often painful bump that develops along the edge of the eyelid. It occurs when an oil gland or hair follicle becomes **infected, typically with staphylococcal bacteria**. Styes are common in children and usually appear suddenly. They may resemble a pimple and sometimes come to a head and drain on their own.

Causes

- Bacterial infection (most commonly *Staphylococcus aureus*)
- Poor eyelid hygiene or rubbing the eyes with dirty hands
- Blocked oil glands in the eyelid
- Increased frequency during colds or upper respiratory infections

Signs & Symptoms of a Stye:

- A painful, red bump near the edge of the eyelid (upper or lower)
- Localized swelling, warmth, or tenderness
- Mild tearing or a feeling of something in the eye
- Possible crusting of the eyelid
- May be accompanied by mild sensitivity to light or blurred vision if swelling is significant
- Usually affects one eye

Seek Immediate Medical Attention

Seek care if the stye becomes swollen, spreads beyond the eyelid, or interferes with vision. A stye that does not improve within 5–7 days, recurs frequently, or is accompanied by fever or excessive tearing should also be evaluated. Medical intervention is advised if your child has difficulty opening the eye or the eyelid appears severely inflamed or discolored.

Natural Remedies for Stye Relief

1. Chamomile Tea Compress

Rationale:

Chamomile has natural anti-inflammatory and soothing effects. When used as a warm compress, it may help reduce swelling and support drainage of a stye.

Instructions:

a. Steep 1 chamomile tea bag in hot water for 5 minutes.
b. Let the tea bag cool to a safe, warm temperature.
c. Place the damp tea bag over the closed eyelid for 5–10 minutes.
d. Repeat 2–3 times daily using a new tea bag each time.

Precaution:

- For external use only.
- Discontinue if the child has ragweed or chamomile allergies.

2. Colloidal Silver Spray (External Use Only, Age 2+)

Rationale:

Colloidal silver has natural antimicrobial properties and may help reduce bacterial irritation when applied cautiously around the outer eyelid.

Instructions:

a. Lightly mist or dampen a clean cotton pad with colloidal silver.
b. Gently wipe the external eyelid margin—avoiding the inner eye.
c. Apply once or twice daily during active irritation.

Precaution:

- Do not apply directly into the eye.
- Use only pediatric-safe, high-quality colloidal silver products for short-term use.
- Discontinue if redness or swelling increases.

3. Coconut Oil

Rationale:

Coconut oil offers soothing anti-inflammatory and gentle antimicrobial benefits. Applying to the skin near the stye may help reduce irritation and limit bacterial spread.

Instructions:

a. Use a clean cotton swab to apply a thin layer of organic virgin coconut oil to the external eyelid margin.
b. Apply 1–2 times daily until symptoms resolve.
c. Use only on intact skin.

Precaution:

- Do not apply coconut oil directly into the eye.
- Discontinue use if redness or irritation worsens.

4. Warm Compress

Rationale:

A warm compress helps open blocked oil glands, promotes circulation, and encourages natural drainage of a stye. This may reduce discomfort and support faster healing.

Instructions:

a. Soak a clean washcloth in warm (not hot) water and wring out excess liquid.
b. Gently place the cloth over the closed eyelid for 10–15 minutes.

c. Repeat 3–4 times daily, using a fresh cloth for each session.
d. Allow the stye to drain naturally—do not squeeze or pop.

Precaution:

- Test water temperature before applying to ensure it's safe.
- Do not reuse washcloths between treatments to avoid spreading bacteria.

Chalazion (Eyelid Cyst)

A **chalazion** is a painless, firm bump on the eyelid caused by a **blocked meibomian (oil) gland**. Unlike a stye, which is an active bacterial infection, a chalazion is **non-infectious** and often develops more gradually. It may persist for weeks but typically resolves on its own with supportive care.

Causes

- Blocked or inflamed oil glands in the eyelid
- Previous stye or chronic eyelid inflammation
- Poor eyelid hygiene
- Skin conditions like seborrheic dermatitis or rosacea

Signs & Symptoms of Chalazion

- Firm, painless lump on the upper or lower eyelid
- Mild eyelid swelling or redness
- Heaviness or pressure sensation in the eyelid
- Sometimes mild tearing or blurred vision if the chalazion presses on the eyeball
- Usually not tender unless it becomes secondarily infected.

Seek Immediate Medical Attention

- Persists for longer than 2-3 weeks
- Grows large enough to affect vision
- Becomes painful or red (may indicate infection)
- Reoccurs frequently
- Is accompanied by a fever.

Natural Remedies for Chalazion

1. Coconut Oil (Topical)

Rationale:

Coconut oil has natural anti-inflammatory and antimicrobial properties that may help calm irritation and support healing of the skin around a chalazion.

Instructions:

a. Dip a clean cotton swab into organic virgin coconut oil.
b. Apply a thin layer to the external eyelid, avoiding the eye itself.
c. Use 1–2 times daily, especially after cleansing or warm compresses.

Precaution:

- Do not apply directly into the eye or inner eyelid.
- Discontinue use if irritation or redness worsens.

2. Eyelid Massage

Rationale:

Gentle massage after warming the area can promote drainage of the blocked gland and speed up the resolution of the chalazion.

Instructions:

a. Always follow a warm compress with clean hands.
b. Use a fingertip to gently massage the closed eyelid in small circular motions.
c. Focus on the area near the lump using light, steady pressure.
d. Massage for 1–2 minutes once or twice per day.

Precaution:

- Do not apply direct pressure over the lump.
- Stop massage if the eyelid becomes painful or inflamed.

3. Lid Hygiene

Rationale:

Regular cleaning of the eyelid and lashes removes oil, bacteria, and debris, helping prevent new or recurring chalazia.

Instructions:

a. Mix 1 drop of tear-free baby shampoo or gentle eyelid cleanser in ½ cup of warm water.
b. Soak a clean cotton pad or gauze in the solution.
c. Gently clean along the lash line of the affected eye.
d. Rinse with warm water and pat dry. Perform daily during flare-ups or as prevention.

Precaution:

- Avoid allowing cleanser to enter the eye.
- Discourage eye rubbing and ensure clean hands before touching the face.

4. Warm Compress

Rationale:

Applying a warm compress softens hardened oil, improves blood flow, and encourages drainage of the blocked gland, helping the chalazion resolve more quickly.

Instructions:

a. Soak a clean washcloth in warm (not hot) water and wring out the excess.
b. Gently place over the closed eyelid for 10–15 minutes.
c. Repeat 3–4 times daily using a fresh cloth each time.

d. Continue daily until the lump reduces in size or resolves.

Precaution:

- Always check that the cloth is warm, not hot, to avoid burns.
- Do not attempt to squeeze or pop the lump.
- Use a clean cloth for each session to reduce contamination.

Foreign Object in the Eye

Foreign objects in the eye are a common concern in infants and children and may include dust, dirt, eyelashes, sand, or small debris. While most small particles cause only temporary irritation, some can lead to **scratching, infection, or more serious damage** if not handled properly. Prompt, gentle care is essential.

Causes

- Outdoor play or wind-blown particles
- Contact with sand, dirt, or dust
- Accidental touch or rubbing of the eyes
- Small insects or airborne debris
- Cosmetics or soap residue during bathing

Signs & Symptoms of a Foreign Object in the Eye:

- Excessive tearing or watery eyes
- Redness or irritation
- Frequent blinking or squinting
- Rubbing at the eye or visible discomfort
- Sensation of something being "in the eye"
- Light sensitivity or mild swelling
- Visible particle under eyelid or on eye surface

Seek Immediate Medical Attention

- The object is embedded or cannot be removed easily
- The child has **vision changes** or **persistent light sensitivity**
- There is **bleeding**, pus, or discharge from the eye
- Pain continues despite flushing
- **The object is sharp, chemical-based, or caused by high-impact trauma**
- **The child is unable to open the eye** or becomes inconsolable

Safe Removal Techniques for Minor Foreign Objects

1. *Sterile Saline or Water Flush*

Rationale:

Rinsing with sterile solution helps **gently remove irritants** and debris without rubbing or increasing the risk of abrasion.

Instructions:

a. Wash your hands thoroughly.
b. Use sterile saline eye drops or **boiled, cooled water** in a clean dropper or syringe.
c. Tilt the child's head to the side so fluid drains outward.
d. Gently flush the eye starting from the inner corner outward.
e. Allow the child to blink several times to help dislodge the object.
f. Repeat as needed, using only sterile solution and clean supplies.

2. *Blinking Method*

Rationale:

Blinking stimulates natural tear production, which may help **wash out small, loose particles**.

Instructions:

a. Encourage the child to blink repeatedly if cooperative.
b. Avoid rubbing the eye, which may cause scratching.
c. If irritation persists after blinking and tearing, proceed with a saline rinse.

3. Cotton-Tipped Swab (visible on surface)

Rationale:

A soft, moistened swab can sometimes **lift a visible particle** from the eyelid or lash line safely if it does not move with blinking or rinsing.

Instructions:

a. Only attempt this if the object is clearly visible and easily reachable.
b. Use a clean, damp cotton swab or sterile gauze.
c. Gently touch the edge of the object to lift it out, avoiding direct contact with the eye surface.
d. Never use fingernails, sharp tools, or apply pressure.

4. Do Not Rub or Apply Pressure

Rationale:

Rubbing the eye can **push debris deeper**, scratch the cornea, or increase risk of infection.

Instructions:

a. Keep the child's hands clean and gently discourage rubbing.
b. Use a cool compress if needed for comfort.
c. If discomfort persists, keep the eye closed and seek medical evaluation.

Head Lice

What Are Head Lice?

Head lice are tiny, wingless, parasitic insects that live on the scalp and feed on human blood. They are common in children and spread primarily through direct head-to-head contact, not through poor hygiene. Lice are not dangerous, but they can cause itching, irritation, and social discomfort.

How to Identify Head Lice on a Child:

- Itching: The most common early sign is persistent scratching of the scalp, especially behind the ears and at the nape of the neck.
- Nits (eggs): Tiny white or yellowish oval-shaped eggs attached firmly to hair strands, often near the scalp. They do not flake off like dandruff.
- Live lice: Small, tan or gray insects (about the size of a sesame seed) that move quickly when exposed to light. They can be hard to spot.
- Red bumps or scratch marks: Especially along the neckline or scalp from scratching.
- Irritability or trouble sleeping: Lice are more active at night and may disrupt sleep.

A fine-toothed lice comb is the best tool to detect both live lice and nits. Part the hair into small sections and inspect closely under bright light.

Natural Remedies & Home Care for Lice

1. Cleaning & Environmental Control

Rationale:

While lice do not live long off the scalp, cleaning bedding, clothing, and hair accessories is crucial to prevent reinfestation.

Instructions:

a. Wash all recently used bedding, hats, and clothes in hot water and dry on high heat.
b. Vacuum upholstered furniture, rugs, and car seats thoroughly.
c. Soak combs and brushes in hot water (at least 130°F) for 10 minutes.
d. Seal non-washable items in plastic bags for 48 hours to starve lice.

Precaution:

- Avoid using pesticide sprays on furniture or bedding.
- Continue cleaning for several days after the last lice sighting.

2. Coconut Oil

Rationale:

Coconut oil can suffocate lice, loosen nits from hair strands, and soothe scalp irritation caused by scratching.

Instructions:

a. Warm (not hot) organic virgin coconut oil and apply generously to the scalp and hair.
b. Cover the head with a shower cap and leave on for 2–3 hours.
c. Follow with wet combing and then rinse thoroughly with shampoo.
d. Repeat every 3–5 days as needed until lice are no longer present.

Precaution:

- Use a towel to catch oil drips.
- Avoid if there is a known coconut allergy.

3. Essential Oil Blend (Ages 2+)

Rationale:

Essential oils like tea tree, neem, lavender, and eucalyptus have natural insect-repelling and lice-killing properties.

Instructions:

a. Mix 2–3 drops of essential oil with 2 tablespoons of a carrier oil (e.g., coconut, olive, or almond oil).
b. Apply to the scalp and hair, then cover with a shower cap for 30–60 minutes.
c. Rinse well and follow with wet combing.
d. Always patch test before full application.

Precaution:

- Not for use in children under age 2.
- Avoid contact with eyes, nose, and mouth.
- Discontinue if rash or irritation develops.

4. Lice Prevention Spray

Rationale:

Natural repellent sprays can reduce the risk of lice transmission during outbreaks or after exposure.

Instructions:

a. In a spray bottle, combine 10 drops of tea tree oil, 5 drops of lavender oil, and 1 cup of distilled water.
b. Shake well before each use.
c. Lightly spray onto dry hair each morning before school or group activities.

Precaution:

- Avoid spraying near the eyes or face.
- Store in a cool, dark place and label clearly.
- Discontinue if sensitivity occurs.

5. *Peppermint Oil in Shampoo (Preventative Use)*

Rationale:

Peppermint oil's strong scent overwhelms lice and discourages attachment, making it useful as a preventative during lice outbreaks.

Instructions:

a. Add 5–10 drops of peppermint essential oil to an 8 oz bottle of unscented or child-safe shampoo.
b. Mix thoroughly and label the bottle clearly.
c. Use during regular hair washing, especially during lice outbreaks.

Precaution:

- Do not use in children under age 2.
- Avoid contact with eyes.
- Patch test before first use.

6. *Wet Combing Method (Mainstay of Natural Treatment)*

Rationale:

Wet combing physically removes lice and nits without the use of chemicals. It is safe for all ages and essential for effective lice removal.

Instructions:

a. Apply thick conditioner or natural oil (e.g., coconut or olive oil) to damp hair.
b. Section the hair and comb from scalp to ends using a fine-toothed lice comb.
c. Wipe the comb on a tissue after each pass and inspect for lice or nits.
d. Repeat every 3–4 days for at least 2 weeks or until no lice or nits remain.

Precaution:

- Clean combs between uses.
- Ensure good lighting for accurate inspection.

Cradle Cap (Infant Seborrheic Dermatitis)

Cradle cap is a common, harmless skin condition seen in infants, typically appearing in the **first few weeks of life**. It causes **scaly, greasy patches on the scalp**, and can also affect the **forehead, eyebrows, behind the ears**, and **upper neck**. Though it may look concerning, it usually doesn't cause discomfort and is not contagious.

Causes

- Overactive sebaceous (oil) glands stimulated by maternal hormones
- Yeast (Malassezia) present on the skin
- Mild inflammation or imbalance in skin microbiota
- Infrequent washing or shampooing may allow buildup

Signs & Symptoms of Cradle Cap

- Flaky, yellow, or white greasy scales on the scalp
- Mild redness or irritation under the scales
- Patches that may spread to eyebrows, ears, or neck
- No itchiness or pain (unlike eczema)
- Hair may appear matted or clumped in affected areas

Seek Immediate Medical Attention

- The scalp becomes **red, swollen**, or **oozing**
- The rash spreads rapidly or shows signs of infection
- The baby appears uncomfortable, is scratching, or losing hair
- Symptoms persist beyond **12 months** or worsen despite home care

Natural Remedies for Cradle Cap

1. Calendula or Chamomile Infused Oil

Rationale:

Calendula and chamomile are soothing botanicals with anti-inflammatory and skin-healing properties that may help reduce redness and promote flake removal.

Instructions:

a. Use a pre-prepared calendula or chamomile-infused oil, or steep dried flowers in a carrier oil like jojoba or olive for several hours.
b. Let cool and strain out the herbs.
c. Apply a small amount to the scalp or affected areas and massage gently.
d. Let sit for 15–20 minutes, then follow with soft brushing and shampooing.
e. Repeat 1–2 times weekly or as needed.

Precaution:

Perform a patch test on a small area before full application. Do not use essential oils directly on infant skin without proper dilution.

2. Coconut Oil Scalp Massage

Rationale:

Coconut oil softens scales, moisturizes dry skin, and provides gentle antifungal support to the scalp.

Instructions:

a. Warm a small amount of organic virgin coconut oil between your hands.
b. Gently massage the oil into the scalp, behind the ears, and on eyebrows if affected.

c. Allow to sit for 15–20 minutes to loosen flakes.
d. Use a soft baby brush to gently lift away flakes.
e. Shampoo afterward to remove excess oil.
f. Repeat 2–3 times weekly as needed.

Precaution:

- Use a gentle baby shampoo to avoid skin irritation.
- Monitor for any allergic reaction or rash.

3. Diluted Apple Cider Vinegar Rinse (Age 3 months+, with pediatrician approval)

Rationale:

Apple cider vinegar (ACV) may help rebalance scalp pH and discourage yeast growth that contributes to cradle cap.

Instructions:

a. Mix 1 part ACV with 3 parts lukewarm water.
b. Using a cotton ball, dab gently onto the scalp, focusing on flaky patches.
c. Allow to sit for up to 10 minutes under supervision.
d. Rinse thoroughly and wash with mild shampoo.
e. Use 1–2 times per week as tolerated.

Precaution:

- Not recommended for infants under 3 months without pediatric approval.
- Avoid contact with eyes or broken skin.
- Discontinue if redness or irritation increases.

4. Gentle Brushing with Soft Baby Brush

Rationale:

Gently loosening flakes after oil treatments allows for natural exfoliation without harming delicate infant skin.

Instructions:

a. After applying coconut oil or botanical oil and letting it sit, use a soft baby brush.
b. Gently massage the scalp in circular motions to lift and remove softened flakes.
c. Avoid excessive pressure or scraping.
d. Rinse with warm water and wash with baby shampoo.

Precaution:

- Do not scrub irritated or broken skin.
- Clean the brush after each use to avoid residue buildup.

Dandruff in Older Children

Dandruff is a **scalp condition marked by flaking and sometimes mild itching**. It is more common in children as they grow older. It is not contagious or dangerous, but it may be cosmetically bothersome or linked to underlying conditions such as **dry scalp**, **seborrheic dermatitis**, or **eczema**.

Causes

- Dry skin or climate changes
- Overgrowth of yeast (*Malassezia*) on the scalp
- Infrequent washing or excessive buildup of oils and dead skin
- Use of harsh shampoos or allergic reactions
- Hormonal changes during puberty

Signs & Symptoms of Dandruff

- White or yellow flakes visible on hair or clothing
- Mild itchiness of the scalp
- Dryness or redness of the scalp
- Greasy or oily patches in more severe cases
- May coexist with scalp sensitivity or eczema

Seek Immediate Medical Attention

See a provider if:

- Dandruff is **not responsive to gentle, natural or medicated treatments**
- The scalp is **painful, cracked, bleeding**, or shows signs of infection
- Dandruff spreads to the **face, neck, or ears**
- There is **hair loss** or scarring

Natural Remedies for Dandruff in Children

1. Aloe Vera Gel (Natural or Store-Bought)

Rationale:

Aloe vera provides soothing, anti-inflammatory benefits and may relieve itchiness and promote healing of irritated scalp skin.

Instructions:

a. Apply a thin layer of pure, alcohol-free aloe vera gel to the clean, damp scalp.
b. Leave on for 10–15 minutes before rinsing, or leave overnight if tolerated.
c. Use 2–3 times per week.

Precaution:

- Ensure the aloe product is labeled safe for skin use and free of added dyes or fragrance.
- Perform a patch test before widespread use.

2. Apple Cider Vinegar Rinse

Rationale:

Apple cider vinegar helps balance the scalp's pH, reduces yeast overgrowth, and removes product buildup that contributes to flaking.

Instructions:

a. Mix 1 part raw, unfiltered ACV with 3 parts lukewarm water.
b. After shampooing, pour the mixture over wet hair and scalp.
c. Let sit for 5 minutes, then rinse thoroughly.
d. Use once weekly as a clarifying rinse.

Precaution:

- Avoid contact with eyes or broken skin.
- Not recommended for use on children under age 3 without professional guidance.

3. Castor Oil for Dandruff

Rationale:

Castor oil is rich in ricinoleic acid, which has anti-inflammatory, antifungal, and moisturizing properties. When applied to the scalp, it can help reduce dandruff caused by dryness, minor fungal imbalances, or scalp irritation. Its thick consistency also helps create a protective barrier and nourishes the scalp.

Instructions:

a. Warm a small amount (1–2 teaspoons) of pure, cold-pressed castor oil by placing the bottle in a bowl of warm water.
b. Part the hair and apply the oil directly to the scalp using fingertips or a cotton ball.
c. Gently massage the scalp for 5–10 minutes to improve circulation and absorption.
d. Leave the oil on for at least 30 minutes or overnight (cover with a soft cap if overnight).
e. Rinse out with a mild, natural shampoo. Two washes may be needed to fully remove the oil.
f. Use once or twice weekly as needed.

Precaution:

- Avoid use on open sores or inflamed scalp conditions unless approved by a healthcare provider.
- Always perform a patch test before first use to rule out allergic reaction.
- Ensure the child does not ingest castor oil.
- For children under 2, consult a pediatrician before topical use.

4. Coconut Oil Scalp Treatment

Rationale:

Coconut oil moisturizes dry scalp, reduces flaking, and contains lauric acid, which offers mild antimicrobial properties.

Instructions:

a. Warm 1–2 teaspoons of organic virgin coconut oil between your hands.
b. Massage gently into the scalp and hair.
c. Leave on for at least 30 minutes, then shampoo to remove residue.
d. Repeat 1–2 times weekly.

Precaution:

- Use only fresh, uncontaminated coconut oil.
- Avoid if the child has a coconut allergy or scalp sensitivity.

5. Tea Tree Oil Shampoo (Age 3+)

Rationale:

Tea tree oil has antifungal and anti-inflammatory effects that target dandruff-causing organisms and relieve scalp irritation.

Instructions:

a. Use a child-safe shampoo that contains diluted tea tree oil, or add 2–3 drops of essential oil to 8 ounces of gentle shampoo.
b. Lather and massage into the scalp, leaving on for 2–3 minutes.
c. Rinse thoroughly and repeat 2–3 times per week.

Precaution:

- Not for use in children under 3 years old.
- Always perform a patch test before use to check for skin sensitivity.

- Avoid contact with eyes and mucous membranes.

Headaches in Children

Headaches in children are common and may range from mild tension-type discomfort to more serious neurological symptoms. They can be caused by **dehydration, stress, eye strain, viral illness, sinus pressure**, or in rare cases, **more serious conditions**. While most headaches in children are not dangerous, it's important to monitor their pattern, severity, and associated symptoms.

Causes

- Tension or stress (common cause in school-aged children)
- Dehydration or hunger
- Eye strain (from screen time or poor vision)
- Sinus congestion or allergies
- Inadequate sleep or irregular routines
- Viral infections (cold, flu, etc.)
- Caffeine withdrawal (in older children who consume soda or chocolate)
- **Rarely:** concussion, increased intracranial pressure, brain infection, or tumor

Signs & Symptoms of Headaches in Children

- Complaints of head pain or pressure (forehead, temples, back of head)
- Irritability, crying, or holding the head (especially in toddlers)
- Sensitivity to light or sound
- Nausea or upset stomach
- Fatigue or changes in behavior
- Difficulty concentrating
- Frequent requests to lie down or rest

Seek Immediate Medical Attention

- Has a **sudden or severe headache** (especially if described as "**the worst ever**")
- Wakes from sleep due to head pain
- Has a headache with **vomiting**, **stiff neck**, **fever**, or **confusion**
- Experiences **vision changes**, **loss of balance**, or **weakness**
- Recently suffered a **head injury**
- Has **frequent or worsening headaches** over time
- Is under the age of 3 and cannot describe symptoms clearly

Natural Remedies & Comfort Measures for Headaches

1. *Acupressure & Pressure Point Relief*

Rationale:

Gentle acupressure stimulates circulation, relaxes muscles, and may trigger natural pain relief. This is especially helpful for stress, sinus, or tension-related headaches.

Instructions:

A. **Third Eye Point (Yintang):**
   a. Press gently between the eyebrows using your index finger.
   b. Hold for 30 seconds, then release.
   c. Repeat 2–3 times.

B. **Base of Skull (Occipital Point):**
   a. Use thumbs to press upward into the hollows beneath the skull ridge behind the ears.
   b. Massage gently in circles for 1 minute, then rest.

C. **Hand Web (Hegu Point):**
   a. Gently squeeze the area between thumb and index finger.

b. Hold pressure for 30 seconds, then repeat on the other hand.

Precaution:

- Do not use hand web point on pregnant individuals.
- Use only gentle pressure suitable for the child's age.
- Avoid causing pain or overstimulation.

2. Cool Compress

Rationale:

A cool compress may help relieve tension and inflammation around the head or neck.

Instructions:

a. Wet a soft cloth with cool water and wring out excess.
b. Apply to the child's forehead or neck for 10–15 minutes.
c. Repeat as needed throughout the day.

Precaution:

- Never apply ice directly to the skin.
- Supervise to prevent cold exposure in younger children.

3. Essential Oils (For Children Over Age 4+)

Rationale:

Lavender and peppermint oils have relaxing and mild analgesic properties that can reduce headache severity.

Instructions:

a. Dilute 1 drop of essential oil in 1 teaspoon of carrier oil.
b. Apply to the temples, back of the neck, or wrists.
c. Avoid the eyes and mucous membranes.

Precaution:

a. Not for use in children under 4.

b. Perform a patch test before full use.
c. Do not use undiluted oils or apply near eyes.

4. Hydration

Rationale:

Headaches are often caused or worsened by dehydration. Adequate fluid intake helps resolve symptoms and prevent recurrence.

Instructions:

a. Offer frequent small sips of water or homemade electrolyte drink.
b. Coconut water or diluted juice may also be used for older children.
c. Avoid sugary or caffeinated beverages.

Precaution:

- Monitor for signs of dehydration: dry lips, sunken eyes, dark urine.
- Encourage fluid intake early during symptoms.

5. Magnesium-Rich Snacks

Rationale:

Magnesium supports nerve and muscle function and may help reduce certain headaches, especially migraines.

Instructions:

a. Offer foods like bananas, avocados, sunflower seeds, or plain yogurt.
b. Keep meal times consistent to avoid low blood sugar triggers.

Precaution:

- Avoid processed or overly salty snacks.

- Consult a provider before using magnesium supplements.

6. *Neck and Shoulder Massage*

Rationale:

Releasing muscle tension in the neck and upper back may help relieve tension headaches and reduce radiating pain.

Instructions:

a. Use gentle circular motions to massage the shoulders and neck.
b. Apply light pressure at the base of the skull.
c. Consider using diluted lavender oil (age 6+) for added relaxation.

Precaution:

- Avoid firm pressure on sensitive or swollen areas.
- Discontinue if discomfort worsens.

7. *Rest in a Dark, Quiet Room*

Rationale:

Sensory reduction can ease headache symptoms, especially in children sensitive to light, sound, or stress.

Instructions:

a. Encourage rest in a quiet, dimly lit or dark room.
b. Provide soft pillows and a calming environment.
c. Allow for a nap or quiet time as needed.

Precaution:

- Avoid screens or loud noises during recovery.
- Monitor for worsening symptoms that disrupt sleep.

CHAPTER 05

RESPIRATORY HEALTH

This section is for educational purposes only. The remedies listed are intended to support comfort and wellness and should not be used as a substitute for professional medical advice. Always consult your child's healthcare provider for diagnosis and treatment.

Warning: Recognizing a Medical Emergency

Shortness of breath can be a ***serious medical emergency****. If a child is experiencing* ***severe, persistent, or worsening difficulty breathing, seek immediate emergency medical care or call 911.***

Signs That Require Immediate Medical Attention:

- Struggling to breathe or gasping for air
- Rapid or labored breathing
- Bluish tint around lips, face, or fingertips (**cyanosis**).
- Chest retractions (skin pulling in between ribs or at the neck while breathing)
- The child assumes a tripod position for relief, characterized by sitting upright while leaning forward and supporting the upper body with the hands placed on the knees or another surface.
- Wheezing or high-pitched noises when inhaling
- Inability to speak in complete sentences due to breathlessness (older children).
- Extreme fatigue or confusion

Disclaimer

This section is for educational purposes only. The natural remedies and recipes provided are intended to support comfort and wellness and are not a substitute for professional medical evaluation, diagnosis, or treatment. Always consult your child's healthcare provider before beginning any new treatment, especially if symptoms persist, worsen, or involve underlying medical conditions.

Emergency Warning:

If your child experiences difficulty breathing, bluish lips or face, altered consciousness, persistent high fever, severe dehydration, or any sudden or alarming symptoms, **call 911 or go to the nearest emergency room immediately**. Prompt medical intervention is essential to ensure adequate oxygenation and prevent serious complications.

Safety Note:

Some ingredients, such as raw honey, carry age-specific risks. **Do not give honey to children under 12 months of age** due to the risk of infant botulism. **ALWAYS consult with your pediatrician or primary care provide before giving to child.**

Before introducing homemade natural cough syrup recipes, it is important to first emphasize the significance of using high-quality honey in natural remedies.

Why Local Raw Honey is Best for Allergies:

When dealing with **seasonal allergies**, using **local raw honey** is one of the most effective natural remedies. Local honey works because it contains trace amounts of local pollen. When consumed regularly, **this pollen acts as a "natural vaccine,"** gradually helping your body build tolerance to the allergens in your environment.

How It Works:

- Local honey contains small amounts of **pollen from flowers and plants in your region**.
- When consumed in small, consistent amounts, it **introduces these allergens to your immune system** in a mild form.
- Over time, your body builds **immunity** to these allergens, reducing **seasonal allergy symptoms** such as sneezing, congestion, and watery eyes.
- **For best results,** take **½ to 1 teaspoon** of **local raw honey** daily, starting a few months before allergy season.

Not All Honey is Created Equal – Avoid Fake Honey!

Many store-bought honey brands are **highly processed and contain little to no real honey**. Some brands mix **cheap fillers like high-fructose corn syrup**, which unnecessarily removes honey's natural health benefits and even spikes blood sugar levels.

How to Spot Fake Honey:

- If the label lists **"high-fructose corn syrup" or "glucose syrup"**, it's not pure honey.
- **Ultra-filtered honey** (clear, without pollen particles) is often stripped of nutrients.
- Real honey **does not dissolve immediately** in water; it sinks before dissolving.
- Pure honey **thickens or crystallizes over time**—if your honey never thickens, it may be diluted.

Buy raw, unfiltered honey from a trusted source, preferably a local beekeeper or farmers' market.

Why Manuka Honey is the Best for Healing

Manuka honey is considered the **gold standard**, though it can be more expensive. This **potent honey from New Zealand** is known for its **high antibacterial, antiviral, and wound-healing properties**.

What Makes Manuka Honey Unique?

- It contains **methylglyoxal (MGO),** a potent compound with **antibacterial and antimicrobial effects**.
- It has a **UMF (Unique Manuka Factor) rating**, which measures its **healing strength**. A UMF **of 10+ or higher** is considered **medicinal grade**.
- It **soothes sore throats, fights bacterial infections, and heals wounds** faster than regular honey.

Best Uses for Manuka Honey:

- **Sore Throats & Coughs:** Take **1 teaspoon daily** to coat the throat and fight bacteria.
- **Wound Healing & Burns:** Apply **directly to cuts, burns, and infections** to speed up recovery.
- **Gut Health:** Helps with **acid reflux, stomach ulcers, and gut bacteria balance**.

Natural Antimicrobial & Cough Support Syrups

Be sure to use organic and whole ingredients to eliminate toxins when possible.

These homemade syrups are designed to support the immune system and ease symptoms of coughs, sore throats, and mild respiratory illness in children. They utilize raw, whole-food ingredients known for their natural antimicrobial, anti-inflammatory, and soothing properties. They can be made at the beginning of a cold or **flu** and stored in a mason jar in the refrigerator for use

1. Elderberry & Clove Cough Syrup

Rationale:

Elderberries contain potent antiviral compounds that support immune function and may shorten the duration of respiratory illness. Cloves provide natural analgesic and expectorant effects, while cinnamon offers antioxidant and antimicrobial support.

Instructions:

a. Combine ½ cup dried elderberries (or 1 cup fresh), 2 cups water, 1 teaspoon cinnamon, and 3 whole cloves in a saucepan.
b. Bring to a boil, then reduce heat and simmer for 30–40 minutes, allowing the liquid to reduce by half.
c. Strain out the solids and let the liquid cool.
d. Stir in ½ cup raw honey and mix thoroughly.
e. Store in a sealed glass jar in the refrigerator for up to 3 months.
f. Administer ½ teaspoon to children over 1 year old every 3 hours during illness or once daily for prevention.

Precaution:

- Never use raw elderberries, which are toxic unless cooked.

- Avoid use in children with known berry allergies.
- Do not exceed the recommended dose.

2. Fire Cider Cough & Immunity Tonic (Age 5+)

Rationale:

This pungent herbal tonic supports immune response, enhances circulation, and relieves sinus and chest congestion. Ingredients like horseradish, garlic, and cayenne help clear mucus, while vinegar and turmeric add antimicrobial and anti-inflammatory effects.

Instructions:

a. In a clean jar, combine ½ cup apple cider vinegar, 1 chopped onion, 3 minced garlic cloves, 1 tablespoon grated horseradish, 1 hot pepper (or ½ teaspoon cayenne), 1 teaspoon turmeric, and the juice of 1 lemon.
b. Allow mixture to sit at room temperature for 24 hours.
c. Strain and discard solids.
d. Stir in ½ cup raw honey.
e. Store in the refrigerator for up to 3 months.
f. Give children age 5 and up ½ teaspoon diluted in warm water once daily or every 4 hours during illness.

Precaution:

- Not suitable for children under age 5.
- Cayenne may irritate sensitive mouths or throats; always dilute.
- Introduce spicy ingredients cautiously and discontinue if discomfort occurs.

3. Ginger, Lemon, and Honey Cough Syrup

Rationale:

Ginger reduces inflammation and soothes throat irritation. Lemon provides immune-boosting vitamin C, while honey coats the throat and offers antibacterial benefits.

Instructions:

a. Boil 2 tablespoons grated fresh ginger in 1 cup of water for 10 minutes.
b. Strain out ginger and cool slightly.
c. Stir in 2 tablespoons lemon juice and ½ cup raw honey.
d. Store in a clean glass jar in the refrigerator for up to 2 weeks.
e. Give children over 1 year old ½ teaspoon every 3–4 hours as needed.

Precaution:

- Do not give honey to children under 1 year.
- Use only fresh, raw ingredients.
- Test for ginger or citrus sensitivity prior to use.

4. Honey, Onion, and Garlic Cough Syrup

Rationale:

Honey offers soothing and antimicrobial properties. Onion and garlic are rich in sulfur compounds that help fight infection, reduce inflammation, and thin mucus.

Instructions:

a. Place 1 small sliced onion and 2 crushed garlic cloves in a clean jar.
b. Cover with ½ cup raw honey and seal.
c. Allow to infuse at room temperature for 12–24 hours.
d. Strain and store the liquid in the refrigerator for up to 2 weeks.

e. Give children over 1 year old ½ teaspoon every 2–3 hours as needed.

Precaution:

- Not suitable for children under 1 year due to honey.
- Discontinue if child is sensitive to garlic or onion.
- Discard if mold or foul odor develops.

5. Pineapple & Turmeric Cough Syrup

Rationale:

Pineapple contains bromelain, a natural enzyme that helps break down mucus and ease coughing. Turmeric reduces inflammation, and honey soothes the throat while fighting microbes.

Instructions:

a. Blend 1 cup fresh pineapple or use pure pineapple juice.
b. Stir in 1 teaspoon turmeric powder, 1 teaspoon grated ginger or ginger juice, and 1 tablespoon raw honey.
c. Mix until well combined and store in a sealed glass jar in the refrigerator for up to 1 week.
d. Give children over 1 year old 1 teaspoon twice daily.

Precaution:

- Avoid use if allergic to pineapple, turmeric, or ginger.
- Shake well before each use.
- Do not use canned pineapple with added sugars.

6. Raw Antimicrobial Syrup with Garlic, Pineapple & Turmeric (Age 2+)

Rationale:

This potent blend uses garlic, onion, ginger, turmeric, pineapple, lemon, apple cider vinegar, and honey to offer natural immune support, reduce inflammation, and ease respiratory discomfort.

Instructions:

a. Peel and chop 1 bulb garlic, 1 small onion, 1–2 inches fresh ginger, and ½ cup fresh pineapple. Place in a glass jar.
b. Add 1 teaspoon turmeric powder and ¼ teaspoon cayenne pepper (optional). Stir.
c. Pour ½ cup apple cider vinegar over the mixture to submerge contents.
d. Let sit for 30–60 minutes at room temperature.
e. Strain and discard solids.
f. Stir in juice of 1 lemon and ½ cup raw honey. Mix well.
g. Store in the refrigerator for up to 3 weeks.
h. Give children age 2 and up 1 teaspoon every 3–4 hours at the first sign of illness. May be diluted in warm water or herbal tea.

Precaution:

- Not for children under age 2 unless supervised by a healthcare provider.
- Omit cayenne for young or sensitive children.
- Always use food-safe tools and clean containers.
- Not a substitute for antibiotics when needed.

Respiratory Support

Supporting a child's respiratory health during illness is essential for their comfort, recovery, and overall well-being. The natural methods that follow are designed to promote open airways, ease congestion, and improve oxygenation through gentle, non-invasive techniques. These remedies encourage better breathing patterns, calm the nervous system, and support the body's innate ability to heal. They are particularly useful during times of respiratory discomfort, such as colds, mild wheezing, or mucus buildup, and can often reduce the need for medication when used appropriately and under supervision. Always ensure that any breathing difficulty is assessed by a healthcare provider when needed.

Positional Strategies for Respiratory Expansion

Note: Shortness of Breath can be a medical emergency. If a child is experiencing severe or persistent shortness of breath, seek emergency medical treatment immediately.

Combining elevation techniques, breathing exercises, and natural remedies can help open the lungs, naturally improve airflow, and make a child more comfortable. Positioning the body correctly reduces airway restriction, improves oxygen exchange, and provides comfort during respiratory distress.

One of the simplest and most effective ways to assist with **shortness of breath** is through **positioning the body** to maximize lung expansion. Elevating the upper body reduces pressure on the diaphragm and allows for better airflow. Here's how to do it correctly:

1. ***Elevating the Upper Body in Bed (For Sleeping or Resting)***

Rational:

Elevating the head and upper body during rest can aid **respiratory comfort** and **function** in several ways. Gravity assists with **mucus drainage**, helping to **prevent** fluid **buildup** in the **lungs** and reducing compression on the diaphragm, making breathing easier. This position also discourages airway collapse, allowing smoother airflow in and out of the lungs. Additionally, head elevation can reduce episodes of acid reflux, which may otherwise trigger asthma-like symptoms or shortness of breath.

Step-by-Step Instructions:

a. Have the child lie on their **back** or **side** in bed.
b. Use **2–3 firm pillows** or a wedge pillow to elevate the upper body at a **30–45 degree angle**.

c. Ensure the head and neck are aligned with the spine and **not bent forward**, which can restrict airflow.
d. Keep the knees slightly bent by placing a small pillow under them for comfort.
e. Encourage slow, **deep breathing** through the nose and mouth to improve oxygen exchange.

2. Sitting in a Forward-Leaning Position (Tripod Position)

Rational:

The upright or tripod position can significantly support respiratory function during episodes of distress. It **opens the airways and allows the lungs to expand more fully**, enhancing oxygen intake. This posture also **encourages accessory muscles**, such as those in the shoulders and neck, to assist with breathing when the diaphragm alone is insufficient. Reducing compression on the lungs makes inhalation easier and more effective. Additionally, this position can **help reduce feelings of panic** by promoting more stable and controlled breathing patterns.

If child is doing this on their own or in need of this position, this is a medical emergency and you should call 911 or take them to the nearest emergency room.

Step-by-Step Instructions:

a. Have the child **sit in a chair** or on the edge of the bed.
b. Place **a sturdy pillow on their lap**.
c. Lean forward, resting **elbows on the knees** or the pillow.
d. Encourage slow, **deep breathing** in through the nose and out through pursed lips.
e. Avoid **slouching too much**—the back should be supported but slightly bent forward.

3. Side-Lying Position (For Severe Congestion or Mucus Buildup)

Rational:

Sleeping or resting with the head elevated can be especially beneficial for children experiencing respiratory symptoms. This position **keeps the airways open and prevents postnasal drip from pooling in the throat**, which can otherwise lead to coughing or irritation. It also **reduces strain on the diaphragm**, making taking deeper, more effective breaths easier. Additionally, elevation **helps facilitate mucus drainage** from congested lungs and sinuses, promoting clearer airways and more restful sleep.

Step-by-Step Instructions:

a. Have the child **lie on their side** rather than flat on their back.
b. Place **a pillow under their head and one behind their back** for support.
c. Keep their **top leg slightly bent** with a pillow between their knees for comfort.
d. Elevate the head slightly **above heart level** to prevent further congestion.

Chest Congestion

Chest congestion in children refers to the accumulation of mucus in the lungs and lower airways, often causing a wet or rattling cough, labored breathing, and discomfort. It commonly follows viral illnesses such as colds or respiratory infections and may also occur with conditions like bronchiolitis or pneumonia.

Causes:

- Viral infections (e.g., RSV, influenza, common cold)
- Postnasal drip leading to mucus accumulation
- Bronchiolitis, pneumonia, or similar respiratory illnesses
- Allergic reactions producing excess mucus

Signs & Symptoms:

In Infants & Toddlers

- Rattling or wet-sounding cough
- Noisy breathing or wheezing
- Fussiness, poor feeding
- Fast or shallow breathing

Older Children May Experience

- Persistent productive cough
- Chest tightness or pressure
- Shortness of breath during activity
- Trouble sleeping due to mucus

Seek Immediate Medical Attention

If your child exhibits any of the following:

- **Bluish lips or fingernails**
- **Grunting, wheezing, or rapid breathing**
- **Chest retractions (skin pulls between ribs with breathing)**

- **High fever with worsening cough or fatigue**
- **Lethargy, difficulty staying awake, or inability to speak in full sentences**

Natural Remedies for Chest Congestion

1. Aromatherapy (Age 2+)

Rationale:

Aromatherapy using essential oils such as eucalyptus, peppermint, or lavender may help ease congestion by opening airways, calming the nervous system, and reducing inflammation.

Instructions:

a. Choose a high-quality, therapeutic-grade essential oil safe for children (e.g., eucalyptus radiata, peppermint, or lavender).
b. Add 2–3 drops of essential oil to a cool mist diffuser filled with clean water.
c. Place the diffuser in the child's room and run for 15–30 minutes, especially during rest.
d. For topical use, dilute 1 drop of essential oil in 1 teaspoon of carrier oil (e.g., coconut or olive oil).
e. Apply to soles of feet or chest (not the face), up to 2–3 times daily.

2. Chest Physiotherapy (Chest PT) for Children

Chest PT is a physical technique used to help loosen and mobilize mucus in the lungs so it can be more easily coughed up or suctioned out. This can be especially helpful during colds, bronchiolitis, pneumonia, or increased lung secretions.

Rational:

- Loosen thick mucus in the airways.
- Promote lung drainage and deeper breathing.

- Reduce the risk of infection and lung complications.

When to Use Chest PT:

- Wet or productive cough
- Difficulty clearing mucus
- Bronchiolitis, pneumonia, cystic fibrosis, or similar conditions
- As directed by your child's pediatrician

When NOT to Perform Chest PT:

- After meals (wait 1–2 hours)
- If the child has fractured ribs or chest trauma
- During active respiratory distress or high fever, unless directed by a provider
- If your child is too irritable or distressed, stop and try later.

How to Perform Chest PT at Home:

- Clean hands and form a soft, cupped hand.
- Optional: infant chest PT cup or soft suction bulb (never a hard object)
- Comfortable flat surface or parent's lap
- Towel or blanket for support.

Step-by-Step Instructions:

a. **Position the Child Properly**
   Choose one of the following postural drainage positions based on your child's age and comfort:

   - **Infants:** Lay the baby across your lap on their tummy with the head slightly lower than the chest.
   - **Toddlers & Older Children:** Have them lie on their stomach on a firm, slightly inclined surface, or sit in your lap leaning forward against a pillow or your chest.

b. **Cup Your Hand**
   Gently form a **cupped hand** (like holding water in your palm). The air cushion between your hand and

the chest wall creates a light thumping that vibrates through the chest.

c. **Percussion Technique**

- Lightly tap the child's **upper back** between the shoulder blades and on the lower lobes (sides of the back, just under the ribs).
- Alternate between both areas. Use a **steady, rhythmic motion**, like gently drumming.
- **Tap for 2–3 minutes per area** or as tolerated.
- Avoid the spine, kidneys, and stomach area.

d. **Encourage Coughing**
After percussion, sit the child up and **encourage coughing or deep breathing**, which helps move the loosened mucus upward.

- If mucus drains to the nose or throat, gentle suction with a nasal bulb may be used for younger children or infants.

e. **Repeat as Needed**

- Perform **2–4 sessions per day**, especially in the morning and before bedtime.
- Always ensure the child is comfortable and warm afterward.

Aftercare & Tips

- Offer fluids afterward to keep the mucus thin.
- Follow with a warm bath or steam to enhance mucus movement.
- Clean your hands and any tools used.

3. *Chest Rub with Essential Oils (Age 3+)*

Rationale:

A natural chest rub made with child-safe essential oils can ease breathing by reducing nasal congestion and calming cough reflexes.

Instructions:

a. Mix 2 tablespoons coconut oil or shea butter with 1–2 drops each of eucalyptus (radiata), lavender, and frankincense essential oils.
b. Rub a small amount onto the chest, upper back, and soles of feet.
c. Apply before bedtime or as needed.
d. Store remaining rub in a sealed container.

Precaution:

- Do not apply near eyes or nose.
- Not for use in children under age 3.
- Perform a patch test before first use.

4. *Diaphragmatic (Belly) Breathing*

Rationale:

This technique strengthens the diaphragm and promotes full lung expansion, improving oxygen intake and helping clear mucus.

Instructions:

a. Have the child lie down or sit with one hand on the chest and one on the belly.
b. Instruct the child to inhale deeply through the nose so the belly rises.
c. Exhale slowly through pursed lips as the belly falls.
d. Repeat for 5–10 minutes once or twice daily or during breathing difficulty.

Precaution:

- Ensure the child is calm and comfortable.
- Stop if dizziness or anxiety occurs.

5. Gentle Movement or Outdoor Air

Rationale:

Light activity and fresh air encourage deeper breathing and support mucus movement in the lungs.

Instructions:

a. Encourage short walks or light outdoor play, weather permitting.
b. Dress appropriately for the weather.
c. Avoid exposure to cold or damp air.

Precaution:

- Avoid strenuous activity during illness.
- Monitor for fatigue or worsening symptoms.

6. Herbal Respiratory Tea (Age 2+)

Rationale:

Herbal teas such as mullein leaf, marshmallow root, and thyme soothe the respiratory tract, loosen mucus, and calm coughs.

Instructions:

a. Steep 1 tsp dried mullein, marshmallow root, or thyme in 1 cup hot water for 10 minutes.
b. Strain well and cool to a warm, safe temperature.
c. Offer 1–2 ounces 2–3 times daily for children over age 2.
d. Sweeten with a small amount of raw honey if desired (for children over age 1).

Precaution:

- Always strain thoroughly.
- Do not give honey to children under age 1.

7. Homemade "Vicks" Vapor Rub (Natural Chest Balm)

Rationale:

This natural balm opens airways and soothes the chest using essential oils and moisturizing bases.

Instructions:

a. Melt ½ cup coconut oil and 2 tbsp beeswax over low heat.
b. Remove from heat and stir in: – 10 drops eucalyptus oil – 10 drops peppermint oil – 5 drops tea tree oil (optional) – 5 drops lavender oil (optional)
c. Pour into a sterile jar and cool until solid.
d. Apply to chest, back, or soles of feet as needed.

Precaution:

- Reduce oil concentrations for children under age 10.
- Avoid the face and broken skin.
- Do not use on infants under age 2 unless directed.

8. Hydration

Rationale:

Adequate fluids help thin mucus and improve its clearance from the lungs and airways.

Instructions:

a. Offer warm liquids like broth, water, or chamomile tea (age-appropriate).
b. Encourage frequent breastfeeding or formula for infants.
c. Avoid sugary or carbonated beverages.

Precaution:

- Avoid honey in children under age 1.
- Monitor intake to ensure adequate hydration.

9. Humidifier Use (Cool Mist)

Rationale:

A cool mist humidifier moistens dry indoor air, helping soothe the airways, reduce irritation, and thin mucus.

Instructions:

a. Place the humidifier several feet from the child's bed.
b. Use distilled or filtered water.
c. Run during naps and overnight.
d. Empty, rinse daily, and deep clean every 2–3 days.

Precaution:

- Avoid warm-mist models due to burn risk.
- Keep the unit clean to prevent mold and bacteria.

10. Mullein Tea

Rationale:

Mullein is rich in mucilage and anti-inflammatory properties, helping to soothe irritated airways and support lung health.

Instructions:

a. Steep 1 tsp dried mullein in 1 cup hot (not boiling) water for 10–15 minutes, covered.
b. Strain thoroughly.
c. Cool to a warm, safe temperature.
d. Offer in small sips to children over age 2, up to twice daily.

Precaution:

- Always strain to remove fine hairs.
- Not for use in children under 12 months.

11. Pineapple Juice or Bromelain Supplement (Age 2+)

Rationale:

Bromelain, found in pineapple, has anti-inflammatory and mucus-thinning properties that can support respiratory health.

Instructions:

a. Offer fresh pineapple juice in small amounts.
b. Consider a pediatric bromelain supplement as directed.

Precaution:

- Avoid in children with pineapple allergy.
- Stop use if stomach upset occurs.

12. Postural Drainage Positions

Rationale:

Using gravity-assisted positions can help drain mucus from the lungs, promoting clearer breathing and better oxygen exchange.

Instructions:

a. Position the child so the chest is elevated above the head (e.g., face down on a wedge or pillow).
b. Maintain position for 10–15 minutes.
c. Gently tap the back with cupped hands to loosen mucus.
d. Alternate positions and follow with coughing or suction.

Precaution:

- Always supervise.

- Stop if dizziness or distress occurs.

13. Pursed-Lip Breathing

Rationale:

This breathing method slows exhalation and helps keep airways open, easing shortness of breath and promoting calm.

Instructions:

a. Instruct the child to inhale slowly through the nose for 2–3 seconds.
b. Have the child purse lips and exhale slowly for 4–5 seconds.
c. Repeat for 5–10 minutes or during episodes of labored breathing.

Precaution:

- Best suited for older children.
- Stop if dizziness or discomfort occurs.

14. Steam Therapy

Rationale:

Steam inhalation helps open nasal and bronchial passages, reduce congestion, and loosen mucus for easier clearance. The warm, moist air soothes irritated airways and can ease coughing and breathing effort. Facial steamers are a great tool for using or filling the bathroom with steam from a hot shower.

Instructions:

a. Boil 2–3 cups of water, allow to cool slightly. Pour into a heat-safe bowl that will not tip over and spill onto the child
b. (Optional) Add 1–2 drops of eucalyptus or peppermint oil for children over age 3.

c. Place the bowl on a flat surface and have the child sit in front of it.
d. Drape a towel over the child's head and the bowl to trap the steam.
e. Supervise the child as they breathe deeply through the nose and mouth for 5–10 minutes.

Precaution:

- **Never leave the child unattended near hot water.**
- Do not use essential oils in children under age 3.

15. Warm Compress on the Chest

Rationale:

A warm compress relaxes chest muscles, increases circulation, and helps break up mucus during congestion.

Instructions:

a. Use a warm, damp cloth, rice sock, or low-heat heating pad wrapped in a towel.
b. Test temperature on your wrist before applying.
c. Place over the chest for 10–15 minutes.
d. Repeat 2–3 times daily as needed.

Precaution:

- Always supervise use.
- Do not place over broken skin or medical devices.
- Discontinue if redness or discomfort occurs.

CHAPTER 06

GASTROINTESTINAL HEALTH

This section is for educational purposes only. The remedies listed are intended to support comfort and wellness and should not be used as a substitute for professional medical advice. Always consult your child's healthcare provider for diagnosis and treatment

Monitoring for Dehydration

During periods of nausea, vomiting, and diarrhea, monitoring your child's hydration status closely is critical. Young children are especially vulnerable to fluid and electrolyte loss, which can quickly lead to dehydration. Always offer small, frequent sips of liquids such as breast milk, water, herbal teas, or oral rehydration solutions. Avoid sugary drinks and fruit juices, as they can worsen symptoms. During times of illness, children may not be interested in food and have no appetite, this is normal. As long as child is staying hydrated and not behaving lethargic, there is no need to be concerned about lack of appetite. However, if child is not drinking or eating, monitor closely for signs of dehydration and seek appropriate care immediately.

Signs of dehydration in children may include:

- Dry mouth and lips
- Decreased urination (no wet diapers for 6–8 hours)
- Sunken eyes or fontanel (soft spot on top of baby's head)
- Cool, mottled hands and feet
- Lethargy or unusual sleepiness
- Crying without tears
- Rapid heartbeat or breathing
- Irritability or listlessness

If any signs are observed or your child cannot keep down fluids, **seek medical attention** promptly. Early intervention is key to preventing more serious complications.

Nausea

Nausea in children is a queasy, unsettled feeling in the stomach that may or may not be accompanied by vomiting. It can result from infections, food sensitivities, travel sickness, emotional upset, or overindulgence. Addressing nausea gently can prevent dehydration and improve comfort.

Causes:

- Viral gastroenteritis ("stomach flu")
- Motion sickness
- Foodborne illness or food sensitivity
- Emotional stress or anxiety
- Medication side effects or supplement irritation

Signs & Symptoms:

In Infants & Toddlers

- Crying or fussiness with hand-to-mouth gestures
- Poor appetite or refusal to eat
- Pale skin or sweating
- Gagging or spitting up

Older Children May Experience

- Complaints of stomach upset
- Excessive saliva or swallowing
- Dizziness or lightheadedness
- Vomiting or dry heaving

Natural Remedies and Comfort Care for Nausea

1. *Activated Black Charcoal*

Rationale:

Activated charcoal binds to toxins and unwanted substances in the gastrointestinal tract. It may help reduce nausea caused by foodborne illness, mild stomach upset, or ingested irritants.

Instructions:

a. Choose a high-quality activated charcoal product labeled for internal use.
b. For children age 2 and older, use ¼ to ½ of a capsule, adjusted by weight.
c. Mix with applesauce, water, or diluted juice.
d. Offer with a spoon or cup and encourage a few sips of water afterward.
e. Administer only once per day.
f. Wait 2 hours before or after other medications or supplements.

Precaution:

- Do not use with suspected intestinal obstruction or severe constipation.
- Avoid use with prescription medications unless cleared by a provider.
- May cause harmless black stools.

2. *Apples or Applesauce*

Rationale:

Apples are gentle on the stomach and contain pectin, which may help soothe digestive upset.

Instructions:

a. Offer peeled apple slices or plain applesauce in small amounts.
b. Best given after vomiting has stopped and fluids are tolerated.

Precaution:

- Avoid giving if vomiting is active.
- Choose unsweetened, unflavored varieties.

3. Aromatherapy (Peppermint or Lemon)

Rationale:

Inhalation of specific essential oils such as peppermint or lemon may ease nausea by stimulating the brain's nausea control center.

Instructions:

a. Add 1–2 drops of essential oil to a diffuser or cotton ball.
b. Place near the child (but not directly on skin or pillow).
c. Use in a well-ventilated room.

Precaution:

- Only use oils labeled safe for children.
- Avoid strong scents in children under 2.
- Discontinue if the scent worsens nausea.

4. BRAT Diet (Bananas, Rice, Applesauce, Toast)

Rationale:

The BRAT diet consists of bland, low-fiber foods that are easy to digest and help restore appetite after nausea or vomiting.

Instructions:

a. Offer BRAT foods once fluids are tolerated without vomiting for at least 1–2 hours.
b. Begin with small portions, such as half a banana or a spoonful of rice.
c. Introduce foods gradually and monitor tolerance.
d. Continue small portions throughout the day as tolerated.
e. Resume normal diet as symptoms improve.

Precaution:

- Not nutritionally complete—use only during short-term recovery.
- Avoid using as a long-term diet.

5. Fresh Ginger Tea

Rationale:

Ginger is known for its anti-nausea and digestive soothing properties, especially for motion sickness or mild stomach upset.

Instructions:

a. Slice 4–6 thin pieces of fresh ginger root.
b. Simmer in 1 cup of water for 10 minutes.
c. Strain and cool to a warm temperature.
d. Add a small amount of raw honey for children over age 1.
e. Offer in small sips throughout the day.

Precaution:

- Do not use honey for children under age 1.
- Use mild strength to avoid stomach irritation.

6. Grape Juice

Rationale:

Grape juice contains antiviral compounds and is gentle on the stomach when diluted.

Instructions:

a. Offer organic grape juice diluted 1:1 with water.
b. Serve chilled and in small amounts.

Precaution:

- Monitor for excess sugar intake.
- Avoid juice if vomiting recurs.

7. Grapefruit Seed Extract

Rationale:

Grapefruit seed extract has natural antimicrobial properties that may help reduce nausea from digestive imbalance or infection.

Instructions:

a. Use a product labeled for internal use and free of additives.
b. For children over 6: Mix 20 drops into 16 oz water.
c. For under 6: Use 5–10 drops in 8 oz water.
d. Stir well and offer in small sips throughout the day.
e. Shake well before use.
f. Never give undiluted.

Precaution:

- Always dilute—never give full strength.
- May interact with medications—consult a provider.
- Discontinue if rash or tingling occurs.

8. Homemade Electrolyte Drink

Rationale:

Hydration is critical during nausea. Electrolyte drinks restore sodium, potassium, and fluid balance.

Instructions:

a. In 4 cups filtered water, mix ¼ tsp sea salt, ¼ tsp baking soda, and juice of 1 lemon.
b. Stir in 1–2 tbsp raw honey (age 1+).
c. Optional: Add orange slices, fresh fruit, or a splash of juice.
d. Serve room temperature or chilled in small sips.

Precaution:

- Not for infants under 2 years unless directed.
- Use honey only in children over 1 year.
- Avoid commercial drinks with dyes/sugar.

9. Marshmallow Root Tea

Rationale:

Marshmallow root contains mucilage, which coats the stomach lining and helps ease irritation and reduce nausea.

Instructions:

a. Place 1 tsp dried marshmallow root in a tea infuser or cup.
b. Pour 1 cup hot (not boiling) water over it.
c. Steep 5–10 minutes and strain well.
d. Cool to room temperature.
e. Offer in small sips; for young children, start with 1–2 tablespoons.

Precaution:

- Strain well to avoid fine herb particles.
- Do not use in children under 12 months.

10. Nux Vomica (Homeopathic Remedy)

Rationale:

Nux Vomica is a gentle homeopathic remedy for nausea related to overeating, stress, or digestive upset.

Instructions:

a. Use 30C potency pellets labeled for children.
b. Give 3–5 pellets under the tongue or water for young children.
c. Dose every 4–6 hours as needed, up to 3 doses/day.
d. Avoid food or drink 15 minutes before/after dosing.
e. Store away from light, moisture, and strong odors.

Precaution:

- Not for prolonged use without guidance.
- Stop if symptoms worsen or last >48 hours.
- Consult provider before use in infants or with medications.

11. Peppermint Oil (Topical)

Rationale:

Peppermint oil soothes the stomach and relieves nausea by relaxing the digestive muscles.

Instructions:

a. Dilute 1 drop peppermint oil in 1 tsp carrier oil (coconut or olive).
b. Rub gently on the child's abdomen in a clockwise motion.

Precaution:

- Do not use near the face in children under age 5.
- Not for use in infants under 2.
- Stop use if irritation occurs.

12. Vitamin B6

Rationale:

Vitamin B6 supports nervous system regulation and may help reduce nausea, especially when related to hormonal or metabolic causes.

Instructions:

a. Check with a pediatric provider before supplementing.
b. Offer B6-rich foods such as bananas, avocados, and oatmeal as tolerated.

Precaution:

- Do not use supplements without medical guidance.
- Avoid high doses unless directed.

Dietary Tips When Managing Nausea:

- Avoid sugary, processed, and dairy foods until fully recovered.
- Offer small, frequent meals with bland, gentle foods (e.g., bone broth, rice, bananas).
- Prioritize hydration with water, herbal teas, or diluted juices.
- Avoid citrus or acidic foods early on, as they can irritate the stomach.

Vomiting

Vomiting is the forceful expulsion of stomach contents through the mouth. It is a common symptom in childhood, often caused by infections, motion sickness, or food intolerance. Persistent vomiting can lead to dehydration and should be monitored closely.

Causes:

- Viral gastroenteritis (stomach flu)
- Foodborne illness or food poisoning
- Motion sickness
- Fever or high heat exposure
- Emotional stress or anxiety
- Food sensitivities or allergies

Signs & Symptoms:

In Infants & Toddlers

- Frequent spit-up turning into forceful vomiting
- Fussiness or crying with arched back
- Refusal to feed
- Lethargy or dry diapers (sign of dehydration)

Older Children May Experience

- Nausea or gagging before vomiting
- Complaints of stomach pain
- Weakness, chills, or sweating
- Dry mouth and decreased urination

Seek Immediate Medical Attention

If your child shows any of the following signs:

- **Vomiting that lasts more than 24 hours**

- **Signs of dehydration (sunken eyes, no tears, dry lips, few wet diapers)**
- **Vomit containing blood or bile (green/yellow)**
- **Lethargy, listlessness, or confusion**
- **Fever over 102°F with vomiting**
- **Severe abdominal pain or swelling**

1. Apples or Applesauce

Rationale:

Apples contain pectin, which may help settle the stomach and reduce nausea or vomiting. Applesauce is gentle and easier to digest during recovery.

Instructions:

a. Use peeled, soft apple slices or plain applesauce.
b. Offer small amounts once vomiting has ceased for at least 30–60 minutes.
c. Avoid added sugars or cinnamon during recovery.

Precaution:

- Do not offer if vomiting is active.
- Use sparingly until fluids are well tolerated.

2. Avoid Triggers

Rationale:

Strong smells, fried foods, or spicy meals may retrigger vomiting in sensitive children.

Instructions:

a. Keep the child in a cool, quiet environment.
b. Avoid cooking odors and strong perfumes.
c. Do not offer sugary, greasy, or spicy foods until fully recovered.

Precaution:

- Watch for reactions to reintroduced foods.
- Maintain a low-stimulation environment when symptoms are active.

3. Black Charcoal

Rationale:

Activated charcoal binds to unwanted toxins and may help when vomiting is caused by food poisoning or mild gastrointestinal irritants.

Instructions:

a. Use a high-quality, food-grade charcoal.
b. For children age 2+, use ¼ to ½ of a capsule mixed into water or applesauce.
c. Offer only once per day and follow with water.
d. Separate from other medications or supplements by at least 2 hours.

Precaution:

- Not for use in children with intestinal obstruction or chronic constipation.
- May interfere with medication absorption.
- May darken stool temporarily.

4. Bone Broth

Rationale:

Bone broth offers hydration, minerals, and gut-healing amino acids during recovery from vomiting and diarrhea.

Instructions:

a. Warm broth to a comfortable temperature.
b. Offer in teaspoons or sips.

c. Increase as tolerated.
d. Use plain, unsalted broth during acute illness.
e. For homemade preparation, see Chapter 10: Immune Support.

Precaution:

- Strain thoroughly for babies.
- Avoid added salt, herbs, or seasonings.
- Store properly and discard if foul-smelling or cloudy.

5. BRAT Diet (Bananas, Rice, Applesauce, Toast)

Rationale:

These bland foods help ease digestion and slowly reintroduce solids after vomiting.

Instructions:

a. Start once the child can hold down fluids.
b. Offer one item in small bites (e.g., banana slice or spoonful of rice).
c. Gradually introduce others through the day.
d. Monitor for tolerance and resume regular diet slowly.

Precaution:

- This diet is not nutritionally complete—use temporarily only.
- Do not force solids if nausea persists.

6. Cold Compress on Back of Neck

Rationale:

Cooling the back of the neck can calm the nervous system and reduce vomiting urges.

Instructions:

a. Wet a washcloth with cool water.

b. Apply to the neck while the child is lying or seated calmly.
c. Leave for 10–15 minutes and repeat as needed.

Precaution:

- Do not use ice directly on the skin.
- Remove if the child feels too cold or shivers.

7. Fresh Ginger Tea

Rationale:

Ginger contains natural antiemetic properties that help relieve vomiting and nausea.

Instructions:

a. Slice 4–6 pieces of fresh ginger.
b. Simmer in 1 cup water for 10 minutes.
c. Strain and cool.
d. Offer in small sips throughout the day.
e. Add honey for children over age 1.

Precaution:

- Not for infants under age 1.
- Use a mild brew to avoid digestive irritation.

8. Ginger Compress on Abdomen

Rationale:

Warm ginger compresses relax abdominal muscles and support digestive relief.

Instructions:

a. Grate 1–2 tbsp of fresh ginger and wrap in cloth.
b. Soak in warm water for 1 minute.
c. Test temperature on wrist.

d. Place over abdomen for 10–15 minutes while resting.
e. Remove if skin becomes red or irritated.

Precaution:

- Never apply while too hot.
- Avoid on broken or rashy skin.
- Supervise use closely.

9. Grape Juice

Rationale:

Grape juice contains polyphenols that may help combat stomach viruses and is well tolerated post-vomiting.

Instructions:

a. Use high-quality, unsweetened grape juice.
b. Dilute 1:1 with water.
c. Offer chilled in small sips after vomiting subsides.

Precaution:

- Excess sugar may irritate the stomach.
- Avoid offering during active vomiting.

10. Grapefruit Seed Extract

Rationale:

This natural antimicrobial may help when vomiting is caused by gastrointestinal infection.

Instructions:

a. Use child-safe, additive-free extract.
b. Age 6+: Mix 20 drops in 16 oz water.
c. Under age 6: Use 5–10 drops in 8 oz water.
d. Shake well and offer in slow sips.
e. Never use undiluted.

Precaution:

- May interact with medications—check with provider.
- Discontinue if rash or tingling occurs.

11. Homemade Electrolyte Drink

Rationale:

Helps prevent dehydration and supports recovery during or after vomiting episodes.

Instructions:

a. Mix 4 cups water, ¼ tsp sea salt, ¼ tsp baking soda, juice of 1 lemon.
b. Add 1–2 tbsp raw honey (age 1+).
c. Add orange slices, fresh fruit, or a splash of juice.

Precaution:

- Not for babies under 2 years.
- Avoid store-bought electrolyte drinks with additives.

12. Marshmallow Root Tea

Rationale:

Soothes the stomach lining and reduces irritation from vomiting.

Instructions:

a. Steep 1 tsp marshmallow root in 1 cup hot water.
b. Strain and cool to warm.
c. Offer in 1–2 tablespoon doses for young children.

Precaution:

- Strain thoroughly.
- Not for infants under 12 months.

13. Nux Vomica (Homeopathic Remedy)

Rationale:

Helpful for vomiting due to stress, food reaction, or overindulgence.

Instructions:

a. Use 30C pellets.
b. Place 3–5 pellets under the tongue or dissolve in water.
c. Use every 4–6 hours up to 3x/day.
d. Avoid food 15 minutes before and after.

Precaution:

- Not for prolonged use without guidance.
- Stop if symptoms persist over 48 hours.
- Not for infants under 1 year without medical advice.

14. Peppermint Oil (Topical)

Rationale:

Peppermint has antispasmodic properties that ease stomach tension.

Instructions:

- Dilute 1 drop peppermint oil in 1 tsp carrier oil (ie. Coconut oil).
- Rub gently over the abdomen in a circular motion.

Precaution:

- Not for use in children under age 2.
- Avoid the face or eyes.
- Stop if any irritation occurs.

15. Probiotics (Powder or Liquid)

Rationale:

Restore healthy gut flora after vomiting, especially post-infection.

Instructions:

a. Use refrigerated pediatric drops or powder.
b. Add to breast milk, water, or applesauce after vomiting has stopped.
c. Store probiotics in a cool, dark place—preferably refrigerated.

Precaution:

- Avoid if vomiting persists.
- Choose high-quality, cold-shipped products.
- Confirm product is appropriate for child's age.

16. Rest and Rehydration Protocol

Rationale:

Resting the digestive tract and hydrating in small amounts improves recovery.

Instructions:

a. Wait 30–60 minutes post-vomiting before rehydration.
b. Offer 1–2 tsp of fluid every 5 minutes (e.g., electrolyte water, tea, breast milk).
c. Increase gradually as tolerated.

Precaution:

- Avoid large volumes early on.
- Monitor for dehydration signs.

Diarrhea

Diarrhea is characterized by frequent, loose, or watery stools and may be accompanied by cramping, urgency, or abdominal discomfort. It can result from viral or bacterial infections, food intolerances, medication reactions, or gastrointestinal disorders. In children, diarrhea requires close attention due to the risk of dehydration.

Causes:

- Viral infections (e.g., rotavirus, norovirus)
- Bacterial infections (e.g., Salmonella, E. coli)
- Food intolerances or allergies
- Reaction to antibiotics or other medications
- Parasites
- Poor sanitation or contaminated food/water

Signs & Symptoms:

In Infants & Toddlers:

- Frequent loose or watery stools
- Diaper rash or skin irritation
- Fussiness or crying during bowel movements
- Poor feeding or appetite
- Decreased urine output

Older Children May Experience:

- Sudden onset of watery stools
- Cramping or abdominal discomfort
- Urgency to use the bathroom
- Nausea or mild fever
- Fatigue

Seek Immediate Medical Attention

- **Diarrhea lasting more than 48–72 hours**

- **Signs of dehydration: dry mouth, no tears, sunken eyes, no urination for 6–8 hours**
- **Blood or mucus in the stool**
- **High persistent fever**
- **Lethargy or decreased responsiveness**
- **Diarrhea in infants under 6 months of age**

Natural Remedies for Diarrhea

1. Avoid Irritants

Rationale:

Certain foods and drinks may worsen diarrhea by irritating the digestive tract or drawing more water into the intestines.

Instructions:

a. Eliminate processed foods, sugary snacks, and soda.
b. Avoid dairy products except for breast milk.
c. Reintroduce bland foods only after stools begin to firm.

Precaution:

- Avoid offering acidic juices or spicy meals.
- Slowly reintroduce solid foods to avoid relapse.

2. Blueberry Soup or Dried Blueberries

Rationale:

Blueberries are rich in tannins and antioxidants, which help reduce intestinal inflammation, support gut repair, and slow down stool frequency.

Instructions:

a. Simmer a small handful of dried blueberries in just enough water to cover them for 10–15 minutes.
b. Cool the mixture to room temperature.

c. Serve in small spoonfuls to children over 1 year old.
d. Older children may chew dried blueberries slowly, in moderation.

Precaution:

- Avoid whole dried fruit for children under age 3 due to choking risk
- Discontinue use if allergic reactions occur.

3. BRAT Diet (Bananas, Rice, Applesauce, Toast)

Rationale:

These bland foods help ease digestion and slowly reintroduce solids after vomiting.

Instructions:

a. Start once the child can hold down fluids.
b. Offer one item in small bites (e.g., banana slice or spoonful of rice).
c. Gradually introduce others through the day.
d. Monitor for tolerance and resume regular diet slowly.

Precaution:

- This diet is not nutritionally complete—use temporarily only.
- Do not force solids if nausea persists.

4. Carrot Soup

Rationale:

Carrots contain pectin, a soluble fiber that helps firm stools. Carrot soup is nourishing and easy to digest, especially during recovery.

Instructions:

a. Peel and chop 2–3 medium carrots.

b. Simmer in water until soft (15–20 minutes).
c. Blend the carrots and cooking water until smooth.
d. Add a pinch of sea salt to support electrolyte balance.
e. Serve warm in small spoonfuls.

Precaution:

- Ensure the soup is not too hot before serving.
- Avoid adding dairy, butter, or seasoning during active diarrhea.

5. Chamomile Tea

Rationale:

Chamomile soothes the digestive tract with its antispasmodic and anti-inflammatory properties, helping reduce cramping and discomfort.

Instructions:

a. Steep 1 teaspoon dried chamomile in hot (not boiling) water for 5–10 minutes.
b. Strain and cool to room temperature.
c. Offer in small sips throughout the day.
d. For infants over 6 months, give 1–2 teaspoons at a time.

Precaution:

- Not for infants under 6 months.
- Use only pure chamomile labeled for consumption.

6. Diaper Care and Skin Protection

Rationale:

Frequent stools can cause diaper rash. Protecting the skin helps prevent irritation and promotes healing.

Instructions:

a. Gently clean the area with warm water and a soft cloth.

b. Pat dry thoroughly or let air-dry.
c. Apply a natural barrier cream (e.g., zinc oxide, calendula, or tallow balm).
d. Change diapers as soon as they are soiled.
e. Allow brief diaper-free time to let skin breathe.

Precaution:

- Avoid fragranced wipes and harsh soaps.
- Discontinue any cream that causes redness or rash.

7. Homemade Electrolyte Drink

Rationale:

Helps prevent dehydration and supports recovery during or after vomiting episodes.

Instructions:

a. In 4 cups filtered water, mix ¼ tsp sea salt, ¼ tsp baking soda, and juice of 1 lemon.
b. Stir in 1–2 tbsp raw honey (age 1+).
c. Optional: Add orange slices, fresh fruit, or a splash of juice.
d. Serve room temperature or chilled in small sips.

Precaution:

- Not for infants under 2 years unless directed.
- Use honey only in children over 1 year.
- Avoid commercial drinks with dyes/sugar.

8. Hydration

Rationale:

Diarrhea rapidly depletes fluids and electrolytes. Ongoing hydration helps prevent dehydration and supports recovery.

Instructions:

a. Offer small sips of oral rehydration solution (ORS) or homemade electrolyte drink every 5–10 minutes.
b. Breastfed infants should continue nursing frequently.
c. Avoid soda, fruit juices, or sugary drinks.

Precaution:

- Monitor urine output and signs of dehydration.
- If child refuses to drink, seek medical advice promptly.

9. Mashed Potatoes (Plain)

Rationale:

Plain mashed potatoes are a gentle, starchy food that helps absorb excess fluid in the gut and provide energy.

Instructions:

a. Boil peeled white potatoes until soft.
b. Mash with a small amount of cooking water and a pinch of salt.
c. Serve warm in small spoonfuls.
d. Gradually increase amount as tolerated.

Precaution:

- Avoid butter, milk, or oil during active diarrhea.
- Watch for worsening symptoms after reintroduction.

10. Probiotics

Rationale:

Probiotics restore healthy gut flora, reduce inflammation, and may shorten the duration of diarrhea.

Instructions:

a. Choose a refrigerated, multi-strain pediatric probiotic.
b. Mix into breast milk, water, or applesauce.
c. Give once or twice daily after vomiting stops.

Precaution:

- Do not mix with hot liquids.
- Stop use if bloating, rash, or discomfort occurs.

11. Rest and Digestive Reset

Rationale:

Resting the digestive system helps the gut heal and regulate bowel movements.

Instructions:

a. Encourage quiet rest.
b. Hold off on solids during the first few hours of diarrhea.
c. Resume bland foods gradually as symptoms improve.

Precaution:

- Avoid vigorous activity during active illness.
- Reintroduce food slowly to prevent relapse.

12. Slippery Elm Bark Powder

Rationale:

Slippery elm forms a soothing gel that coats the intestines, reducing irritation and supporting digestive repair.

Instructions:

a. Mix ¼ teaspoon of powdered slippery elm into applesauce or cool water.
b. Offer once or twice daily to children over age 2.

c. Give at least 1 hour apart from medications or supplements.

Precaution:

- Not for children under 2 unless approved by a provider.
- Discontinue if allergic reaction occurs.

13. Warm Compress on Abdomen

Rationale:

A warm compress relieves cramping, improves circulation, and soothes abdominal discomfort.

Instructions:

a. Soak a clean cloth in warm (not hot) water and wring it out.
b. Optionally simmer slices of ginger in water and use this infusion to soak the cloth.
c. Test on wrist before placing on the abdomen.
d. Leave in place for 10–15 minutes.

Precaution:

- Do not use compress if the skin is broken or irritated.
- Always supervise use.

Constipation

Constipation in children is defined as infrequent, hard, or difficult-to-pass stools, often accompanied by abdominal discomfort or bloating. While normal bowel patterns vary, most children should have at least one comfortable bowel movement every 1–2 days. Constipation can be functional (no clear medical cause) or secondary to diet, dehydration, emotional stress, or medication.

In Infants & Toddlers

- Straining or crying during bowel movements
- Hard, pellet-like stools
- Less frequent stools (fewer than 3 times per week)
- Bloating or firm belly
- Reduced appetite
- Fussiness or irritability

Older Children May Experience

- Abdominal discomfort or cramping
- Skipping bowel movements for days
- Pain during bowel movements
- Soiling or skid marks in underwear
- Fear of using the bathroom
- Stool withholding behavior

Differentiation from Other GI Issues:

- Chronic constipation often leads to secondary symptoms like bedwetting, urinary frequency, or abdominal pain
- **Encopresis (soiling)** results when soft stool leaks around impacted stool
- If accompanied by **vomiting, weight loss, or severe pain**, further evaluation is warranted

Seek Immediate Medical Treatment

- No bowel movement for more than 5–7 days
- Blood in the stool (not from a visible fissure)
- Vomiting with a distended or painful belly
- Weight loss or poor appetite
- Sudden change in bowel habits with no clear cause
- Recurrent or worsening encopresis or urinary symptoms
- Concern for a structural, neurological, or metabolic disorder

Natural Remedies and Home Care for Constipation:

1. Abdominal Massage

Rationale:

Gentle massage stimulates intestinal movement, relieves gas, and promotes natural bowel activity.

Instructions:

a. Warm a small amount of coconut or olive oil in your hands.
b. Gently massage the belly in a clockwise direction, starting at the lower right, moving up, across, and down.
c. Continue for 3–5 minutes.
d. Repeat 1–2 times daily, especially after meals or before bed.

Precaution:

- Avoid massage during fever, unexplained abdominal pain, or distention.
- Stop if the child shows signs of discomfort.

2. Aloe Vera Juice

Rationale:

Aloe vera has mild laxative effects and may soothe inflammation in the digestive tract.

Instructions:

a. Use only food-grade, decolorized aloe vera juice.
b. For children over age 4, mix 1–2 teaspoons with water or juice.
c. Offer once daily as needed.

Precaution:

- Consult a pediatrician before using.
- Do not use in children under age 4.
- May cause diarrhea or cramping in some children.

3. Apples (With Skin)

Rationale:

Apples provide fiber, sorbitol, and pectin, all of which promote regularity.

Instructions:

a. Wash and slice an organic apple with the skin.
b. Serve in the morning or mix into oatmeal or nut butter.

Precaution:

- Do not peel unless needed for texture.

4. Castor Oil Pack

Rationale:

Castor oil promotes circulation and can support gentle digestive stimulation when applied topically.

Instructions:

a. Soak a flannel cloth in warm castor oil.
b. Place on the child's abdomen, avoiding direct skin contact with oil.
c. Cover with plastic wrap and a warm towel.
d. Leave on for 15–20 minutes while supervised.

Precaution:

- Not for use in children under age 4.
- Always consult with a provider before use.
- Do not apply to broken or sensitive skin.

5. *Chia Seeds*

Rationale:

Chia seeds absorb water and form a gel that helps soften stool.

Instructions:

a. Soak ½ tsp in water for 30 minutes.
b. Mix into a smoothie, applesauce, or yogurt.

Precaution:

- Ensure the child drinks adequate fluids to prevent thickening in the gut.
- Not for children under 2 years.

6. *Daily Toilet Routine*

Rationale:

A regular toilet schedule trains the body's natural rhythm and reduces withholding.

Instructions:

a. Have the child sit on the toilet for 5–10 minutes after meals.

b. Use a footstool to support a squatting position.
c. Encourage relaxation and avoid pressure to "go."

Precaution:

- Make the routine stress-free and age-appropriate.

7. Diet Elimination (If Chronic)

Rationale:

Removing common food triggers like dairy or gluten can help if constipation is chronic.

Instructions:

a. Eliminate one or two common triggers (e.g., dairy, gluten) for 2–3 weeks.
b. Track symptoms and reintroduce one food at a time.
c. Consult a healthcare provider before and during the trial.

Precaution:

- Never eliminate major food groups long term without supervision.

8. Digestive Essential Oil Massage

Rationale:

Certain essential oils, like diluted ginger or fennel, may support digestion and ease constipation when applied topically.

Instructions:

a. Dilute 1 drop of fennel or ginger essential oil in 1 tsp of carrier oil.
b. Gently massage in a clockwise motion on the abdomen.

Precaution:

- Not for infants under age 2.

- Avoid use near the face.
- Always patch test and discontinue if irritation occurs.
- Consult your provider before use.

9. Fennel Tea

Rationale:

Fennel has antispasmodic properties and may reduce gas and help with stool passage. Consult your pediatrician before using.

Instructions:

a. Steep ½ tsp fennel seeds in 1 cup of hot water for 10 minutes.
b. Cool to room temperature.
c. Offer 1–2 teaspoons to infants over 6 months or small sips to older children.

Precaution:

- Use only pure fennel seed labeled for consumption.
- Do not use in children with fennel allergies.

10. Flaxseed (Ground)

Rationale:

Flaxseed provides bulk and mucilage to promote smooth bowel movements.

Instructions:

a. Soak ½ tsp in water overnight.
b. Mix into oatmeal, applesauce, or yogurt.

Precaution:

- Do not use in children under 2 years.
- Must be taken with fluids.

11. Honey (Age 2+)

Rationale:

Honey has mild laxative effects and supports digestive health.

Instructions:

a. Mix 1 tsp of raw honey into warm water or herbal tea.
b. Offer once daily.

Precaution:

- Not for children under 1 due to risk of botulism.
- Use in moderation to avoid excess sugar.

12. Hydration

Rationale:

Water softens stool and supports fiber's action in the gut.

Instructions:

a. Encourage water intake throughout the day.
b. Increase during physical activity or heat.

Precaution:

Avoid excessive juice or soda, which may worsen symptoms.

13. Kiwi

Rationale:

Kiwi contains fiber and enzymes that promote healthy bowel movements.

Instructions:

a. Peel and chop ripe kiwi.
b. Serve alone or blend into a smoothie.

Precaution:

- Watch for allergy if introducing for the first time.

14. Lemon Water

Rationale:

Lemon stimulates bile flow and peristalsis to encourage bowel movement. Can add quality honey for additional benefits to make it more palatable for children if over age of 1.

Instructions:

a. Squeeze half a lemon into a cup of warm water.
b. Offer first thing in the morning to children over age 2.

Precaution:

- Avoid giving to children with citrus sensitivity.

15. Licorice Root Tea

Rationale:

Licorice soothes the digestive tract and may aid gentle relief of constipation.

Instructions:

a. Steep ½ tsp licorice root in 1 cup hot water for 5–10 minutes.
b. Cool and offer in small sips to children over age 4.

Precaution:

- Do not use for more than a few days.
- Not for children with high blood pressure or on steroid medication.
- Consult provider before use.

16. Magnesium Supplements

Rationale:

Magnesium relaxes bowel muscles and draws water into the stool. Consult your pediatrician before use.

Instructions:

a. Use pediatric magnesium citrate or glycinate.
b. Follow dosing on the label or as directed.
c. Offer with water.

Precaution:

- Too much can cause diarrhea or cramping.
- Not for children under age 6 unless advised by a provider.

17. Olive Oil (Extra Virgin)

Rationale:

Acts as a gentle lubricant for the intestines.

Instructions:

a. Give 1 tsp to 1 tbsp to children over age 2 on an empty stomach.
b. May also be added to food.

Precaution:

- Not suitable during active diarrhea.

18. Pear Juice

Rationale:

Pear juice contains sorbitol and fiber and is often better tolerated than prune juice.

Instructions:

a. Use 100% organic pear juice.
b. Offer 1–2 oz once daily to infants over 6 months.
c. Give 2–4 oz to older children.
d. Serve at room temperature or slightly warmed.

Precaution:

- Not for infants under 6 months.
- Excessive intake may cause diarrhea.

19. Physical Activity

Rationale:

Exercise stimulates gut motility and supports digestive rhythm.

Instructions:

a. Encourage 30–60 minutes of daily activity (e.g., walking, play, yoga).

20. Prunes or Prune Juice

Rationale:

Prunes provide sorbitol and fiber for effective constipation relief.

Instructions:

a. Soak 3–4 dried prunes overnight.
b. Serve softened or mashed into food.
c. Dilute prune juice with apple juice (1:1) for children.

Precaution:

- Adjust portion based on age.
- Overuse may cause loose stools.

21. Probiotic-Rich Foods

Rationale:

Foods like yogurt and kefir support gut flora and improve stool consistency.

Instructions:

a. Offer unsweetened yogurt with live cultures.
b. Mix into smoothies or serve with fruit.

Precaution:

- Use only dairy if tolerated.
- Check for hidden sugars or additives.

22. Probiotics (Supplemental)

Rationale:

Restore gut flora balance and reduce inflammation.

Instructions:

a. Choose refrigerated, pediatric-specific brands.
b. Mix into breast milk or soft foods after vomiting subsides.

Precaution:

- Avoid hot liquids.
- Monitor for bloating or rash.

23. Psyllium Husk (Age 6+)

Rationale:

Adds bulk and promotes regularity with sufficient hydration.

Instructions:

a. Mix ½ tsp into water or juice.

b. Drink immediately.
c. Follow with a full glass of water.

Precaution:

- Not for young children.
- May cause bloating if not taken with enough fluids.

24. Squatting Stool

Rationale:

Elevating the feet mimics a natural squatting position, improving bowel alignment.

Instructions:

a. Use a footstool during toilet time.
b. Encourage relaxed posture.

Precaution:

- Supervise younger children.

25. Warm Bath with Epsom Salt

Rationale:

Warm water relaxes abdominal muscles, and magnesium from Epsom salt may be absorbed through the skin to ease bowel function.

Instructions:

a. Fill a warm bath and dissolve 1–2 tbsp Epsom salt.
b. Soak the child for 15–20 minutes.
c. Repeat 1–2 times per week as needed.

Precaution:

- Do not allow the child to ingest the water.
- Avoid if skin is broken or irritated

Constipation in Infants

Constipation in infants differs from that in older children and must be considered in the context of feeding methods and developmental stage.

Exclusively breastfed babies may go several days — sometimes up to a week — without a bowel movement. This can be normal due to breast milk's efficient absorption and utilization.

When it's not a concern:

- Baby appears comfortable and content
- No signs of straining, pain, or excessive gas
- No vomiting or bloating
- Normal feeding patterns and wet diapers

Seek Immediate Medical Treatment

- Baby is unusually fussy or irritable
- Straining or crying during attempted bowel movements
- Abdominal distention or hard belly
- Vomiting or refusal to feed
- No stool for more than 5–7 days without signs of improvement (especially in formula-fed infants)

Natural Supportive Measures

1. *Abdominal Massage*

Rationale:

Gentle abdominal massage helps stimulate bowel activity and ease gas buildup, promoting more regular movements.

Instructions:

a. Warm a small amount of natural oil (coconut or olive oil) in your hands.

b. Gently massage the infant's abdomen in a clockwise motion, following the path of the colon.
c. Continue for 3–5 minutes, especially after feeding or before bath time.

Precaution:

- Do not massage if the infant has a fever, distended belly, or cries in pain.
- Discontinue if signs of discomfort appear.

2. *Bicycle Legs*

Rationale:

Mimicking pedaling helps stimulate the lower abdomen and colon, encouraging bowel movements.

Instructions:

a. Lay the baby on their back on a firm, flat surface.
b. Gently move their legs in a pedaling motion, as if riding a bicycle.
c. Perform for 2–3 minutes several times per day.

Precaution:

Always be gentle and monitor baby's cues. Stop if baby resists or becomes distressed.

3. *Glycerin Suppository (consult your pediatrician)*

Rationale:

Glycerin softens the stool and stimulates a reflex to promote bowel movement.

Instructions:

a. Use an infant-formulated glycerin suppository.

b. Follow the dosage instructions exactly or as advised by your pediatrician.
c. Apply with clean hands and gentle care.

Precaution:

- Use only if directed by a pediatrician.
- Not for regular use—reserved for cases where other remedies have failed.

4. Gripe Water

Rationale:

Specific gripe water formulations include herbs like fennel or ginger, that although may not relieve constipation, it may help relieve gas and digestive issues.

Instructions:

a. Use only gripe water labeled safe for infants and free of artificial additives.
b. Follow dosage instructions on the label.

Precaution:

- Confirm the formula is constipation-supportive, not general colic.
- Always consult your pediatrician before use.
- Not a replacement for hydration or dietary evaluation.

5. Hydration Support (For Older Infants)

Rationale:

Older infants (typically 6+ months) may benefit from additional fluids to soften stools and support digestion.

Instructions:

a. Offer small sips of water (1–2 oz at a time) between feedings if baby is over 6 months.
b. For babies eating solids, offer water alongside meals.

Precaution:

- Do not give water to infants under 6 months unless advised by a doctor.
- Monitor for signs of overhydration (rare, but possible in young infants).

6. *Warm Bath with Epsom Salt (External Use Only)*

Rationale:

A warm bath relaxes the abdominal muscles and may stimulate a natural urge to pass stool.

Instructions:

a. Fill infant's bathtub with warm (not hot) water.
b. Add a small pinch (¼ tsp) of Epsom salt and stir to dissolve.
c. Bathe the infant for 10–15 minutes while gently supporting their back.

Precaution:

- Do not allow baby to ingest bathwater.
- Always test water temperature before placing baby in the bath.
- Avoid Epsom salt if baby has broken or irritated skin.

7. *Warm Compress on Abdomen*

Rationale:

Gentle warmth can help relax intestinal muscles and relieve bloating, promoting bowel movement.

Instructions:

a. Soak a clean washcloth in warm (not hot) water.
b. Wring out and place over the baby's abdomen.
c. Leave for 5–10 minutes while monitoring baby closely.

Precaution:

- Always check temperature on your wrist before applying.
- Never use a heating pad or hot compress on infants.
- Stop if baby becomes red, fussy, or uncomfortable.

CHAPTER 07

URINARY HEALTH

This section is for educational purposes only. The remedies listed are intended to support comfort and wellness and should not be used as a substitute for professional medical advice. Always consult your child's healthcare provider for diagnosis and treatment.

Dehydration and Dark Urine

Dark or concentrated urine in children is often a sign of dehydration, which occurs when fluid loss exceeds fluid intake. This can result from illness (especially fever, vomiting, or diarrhea), high physical activity, or insufficient fluid consumption. Dark urine may also occur temporarily after waking in the morning or with certain foods or vitamins. It is essential to determine the underlying cause.

Urinary Tract Infection (UTI)

A urinary tract infection (UTI) occurs when bacteria enter the urinary tract and multiply, typically in the bladder or urethra. UTIs are relatively common in children, especially girls, and can cause discomfort, behavioral changes, and fever. If untreated, a UTI can spread to the kidneys and cause a more serious infection called pyelonephritis.

Signs and Symptoms of UTI in Children:

- Burning or pain during urination (dysuria)
- Frequent urge to urinate with little output
- Foul-smelling or cloudy urine
- Fever (with or without other symptoms)
- Lower abdominal pain or bladder pressure
- Bedwetting or daytime wetting in a previously trained child
- Irritability or behavioral changes (in infants or toddlers)
- Refusal to eat or drink
- Vomiting or poor feeding (in infants)

Differentiation from Other Urinary Issues:

- Unlike overactive bladder or frequent urination without infection, UTIs typically present with **pain during urination and systemic signs** such as fever or irritability.
- Cloudy or foul-smelling urine is more specific to UTI than most benign urinary issues.

Seek Immediate Medical Treatment

- Fever over 101°F (38.5°C), especially in infants
- Vomiting or refusal to drink
- Blood in the urine
- Back or side pain (suggestive of kidney involvement)
- Lethargy or unusual sleepiness
- Recurrent UTIs or suspected structural abnormality

- UTI symptoms in a child under 2 years of age

Comfort Care and Natural Remedies (Supportive, Not Substitutes for Antibiotics)

1. Avoid Bladder Irritants

Rationale:

Acidic, spicy, or sugary foods can increase bladder inflammation and discomfort, especially during a urinary tract infection.

Instructions:

a. Eliminate citrus fruits, tomatoes, chocolate, carbonated beverages, and artificial sweeteners
b. Offer bland, non-acidic foods such as bananas, oats, rice, and steamed vegetables
c. Gradually reintroduce foods once symptoms resolve.

Precaution:

- Avoid major dietary changes without pediatric guidance.
- Monitor for symptom recurrence after food reintroduction.

2. Colloidal Silver (Short-Term Use, Ages 2+)

Rationale:

Colloidal silver is a natural antimicrobial that may assist with early UTI symptoms by inhibiting bacterial growth.

Instructions:

a. Use only pediatric-specific colloidal silver under healthcare provider guidance.
b. Administer the recommended dosage by dropper or spray, once or twice daily.
c. Use for no more than 3–5 consecutive days unless advised otherwise.

Precaution:

- Not for infants under age 2.
- Avoid long-term use to prevent silver accumulation.
- Discontinue immediately if digestive upset or rash occurs.

3. Corn Silk Tea (Ages 2+)

Rationale:

Corn silk has natural diuretic and anti-inflammatory effects that may relieve burning and urinary discomfort.

Instructions:

a. Steep 1 teaspoon of dried corn silk in 1 cup of hot water for 10–15 minutes.
b. Cool completely before offering.
c. Give 1–2 tablespoons, 1–2 times daily as needed.

Precaution:

- Do not use if your child has a known corn allergy.
- Always ensure the tea is fully cooled to avoid burns.

4. Cranberry Extract or Unsweetened Juice (Ages 1+)

Rationale:

Cranberry contains proanthocyanidins that may prevent bacteria from adhering to the bladder wall, supporting infection prevention.

Instructions:

a. Choose 100% unsweetened cranberry juice or pediatric cranberry extract capsules.
b. Dilute juice with water in a 1:1 ratio.
c. Offer 2–4 oz daily to children over age 1. Capsules may be used in children over age 5 with supervision.

Precaution:

- Not recommended for infants under 12 months.
- Excess consumption may cause stomach upset or diarrhea.
- Avoid in children with cranberry or salicylate allergies.

5. *D-Mannose (Ages 3+)*

Rationale:

D-Mannose is a natural sugar that binds to E. coli bacteria and assists in flushing them out of the urinary tract, particularly useful for bladder infections.

Instructions:

a. Use pediatric powder or chewable forms per label dosing.
b. Mix with water or juice and offer 1–2 times daily during active symptoms.
c. Continue for several days after symptoms improve.

Precaution:

- Not suitable for children under age 3.
- Monitor for loose stools or changes in urination.

6. *Encourage Frequent Voiding*

Rationale:

Regular urination helps flush out bacteria from the urinary tract and reduces the risk of bacterial buildup.

Instructions:

a. Encourage your child to urinate every 2–3 hours.
b. Use gentle prompts or a reward system to support compliance.
c. Avoid withholding urination during school or outings.

Precaution:

- Never pressure a child to void if urination is painful.
- Seek care if pain or refusal to urinate persists.

7. Garlic (Ages 1+)

Rationale:

Garlic has antibacterial and immune-boosting properties that may assist in infection prevention and management.

Instructions:

a. Mix a small amount of freshly crushed garlic into food for children over age 1.
b. For topical use, infuse olive oil with garlic and apply externally over the bladder area (avoid broken skin).
c. Use once daily during acute symptoms.

Precaution:

- Do not give raw garlic alone to young children—it may irritate the stomach.
- Always consult your provider before internal or external use in infants.

8. Hydration with Electrolytes

Rationale:

Adequate fluid intake helps flush the urinary system, while electrolytes support kidney function and prevent dehydration.

Instructions:

a. Offer small sips of filtered water frequently throughout the day.
b. Use a homemade electrolyte drink: mix 1 cup water, ¼ tsp sea salt, 1 tsp lemon juice, and ½ tsp honey and fresh fruits (over age 2).

c. Offer this 1–2 times daily during illness or increased urination.

Precaution:

- Avoid giving honey to infants under 1 year.
- Discontinue if diarrhea or signs of overhydration occur.

9. Increase Fluid Intake

Rationale:

Staying well-hydrated dilutes urine and assists the natural flushing of bacteria from the bladder and urinary tract.

Instructions:

a. Offer filtered water regularly throughout the day.
b. Include diluted herbal teas like chamomile or marshmallow root for children over age 1.
c. Avoid sugary drinks and sodas.

Precaution:

- Infants under 6 months should not be given herbal teas or juice.
- Watch for signs of overhydration in very young children.

10. Marshmallow Root Tea (Ages 1+)

Rationale:

Marshmallow root coats and soothes irritated urinary tract tissues and may relieve burning or discomfort during urination.

Instructions:

a. Steep 1 teaspoon of dried marshmallow root in 1 cup of hot water for 10 minutes.
b. Cool to room temperature.

c. Offer 1–2 tablespoons, up to 3 times daily for children over 1.

Precaution:

- Do not use marshmallow root or related herbs in children with known allergies.
- Ensure proper straining to remove herbal particles.

11. Probiotics

Rationale:

Probiotics restore healthy gut and urinary flora, especially after antibiotics or during recurrent infections.

Instructions:

a. Use a refrigerated, multi-strain pediatric probiotic containing Lactobacillus rhamnosus or L. reuteri.
b. Administer once daily mixed into cool food or liquids.
c. Continue use for at least 1–2 weeks following antibiotic therapy.

Precaution:

- Avoid probiotics in immunocompromised children unless approved.
- Do not mix into hot liquids, which destroy live cultures.

12. Warm Sitz Bath

Rationale:

Soaking the pelvic area in warm water can reduce inflammation and relieve pain or burning after urination.

Instructions:

a. Fill a clean basin or shallow tub with warm (not hot) water to hip level.

b. Have the child sit for 10–15 minutes, 1–2 times daily.
c. Dry the area thoroughly after soaking.

Precaution:

- Always test the water temperature beforehand.
- Discontinue if irritation, rash, or discomfort worsens.
- Do not use with open wounds or active skin infections.

Painful Urination (Dysuria)

Dysuria refers to discomfort, burning, or pain during urination. It is a common symptom in children and can range from mild irritation to an indication of infection or inflammation of the urinary tract or genital area.

Causes

- Chemical irritants (soaps, bubble baths, wipes)
- Tight clothing or poor hygiene
- Dehydration or concentrated urine
- Mild urinary tract infections
- Vaginitis or local skin irritation

Signs & Symptoms

In Infants & Toddlers:

- Crying or arching back during urination
- Decreased urine output
- Fussiness with diaper changes
- Redness around genital area

Older Children May Experience:

- Burning or stinging while urinating
- Urgency to urinate frequently
- Lower abdominal discomfort
- Complaints of genital discomfort

Differentiation from Other Urinary Issues:

- UTIs typically include painful urination plus systemic signs (fever, foul-smelling urine, irritability)
- Chemical irritation (from bubble baths, soaps, or wipes) causes pain without fever or systemic symptoms

- Pinworms may cause itching and burning near the urethra, especially at night

Seek Immediate Medical Treatment

- Painful urination lasting more than 24–48 hours
- Accompanied by fever, abdominal pain, or back pain
- Blood in the urine
- History of recurrent UTIs
- Child is refusing to urinate due to pain
- Symptoms in a child under 2 years old

Comfort Care and Natural Remedies Dysuria:

1. Chamomile or Marshmallow Root Tea

Rationale:

Both herbs have soothing, anti-inflammatory properties that may help calm urinary and bladder irritation internally.

Instructions:

a. For children over age 1, steep 1 tsp dried chamomile or marshmallow root in 1 cup hot water for 5–10 minutes.
b. Cool to room temperature before offering.
c. Offer in small sips throughout the day.

Precaution:

- Do not give to infants under 12 months.
- Ensure the tea is free from added flavors or sweeteners.
- Discontinue if rash or allergy symptoms appear.

2. Coconut Oil or Emu Oil (Topical Use)

Rationale:

These oils provide natural moisture and soothing relief for external genital irritation, especially around the urethral opening.

Instructions:

a. Gently cleanse the area with warm water only and pat dry.
b. Apply a small amount of pure coconut or emu oil to the external area.
c. Use 1–2 times daily after diapering or bathing.

Precaution:

- Do not insert oils internally.
- Discontinue use if rash, redness, or worsening irritation occurs.

3. Eliminate Irritants (Soaps, Bubble Baths, Wipes)

Rationale:

External chemical irritants are a leading cause of dysuria in young children, particularly girls.

Instructions:

a. Use only warm water for cleansing the diaper or genital area.
b. Avoid all perfumed soaps, scented wipes, and bubble baths.
c. Allow the area to air dry when possible.

Precaution:

- Always check product labels for hidden fragrances or chemicals.
- Seek medical advice if symptoms persist despite stopping irritants.

4. *Increase Water Intake*

Rationale:

Flushing the urinary tract with diluted urine may relieve irritation and prevent worsening symptoms.

Instructions:

a. Encourage frequent small sips of water throughout the day.
b. For children over 1 year, small amounts of diluted herbal teas can also support hydration.
c. Avoid citrus, tomato, or carbonated beverages until symptoms resolve.

Precaution:

- Monitor fluid intake closely in young children.
- Limit herbal teas to age-appropriate children and use only under supervision.

5. *Warm Sitz Bath*

Rationale:

Warm water immersion provides external relief from burning, irritation, or inflammation.

Instructions:

a. Fill a shallow basin or tub with warm (not hot) water to cover the child's hips.
b. Do not add soap, essential oils, or bath products.
c. Allow the child to sit in the bath for 10–15 minutes.
d. Pat dry with a soft, clean towel.
e. Repeat 1–2 times daily as needed.

Precaution:

- Always test water temperature to avoid burns.

- Discontinue if skin becomes red, irritated, or if child is uncomfortable.
- Do not use if there are open sores or active rashes.

Bedwetting (Nocturnal Enuresis)

Bedwetting, or nocturnal enuresis, refers to involuntary urination during sleep in a child who is old enough to have bladder control, typically beyond age 5. It is a common pediatric issue and is considered part of normal development unless it persists or causes distress.

Signs and Symptoms

- Nighttime wetting during sleep, usually in the early hours of the night or morning
- No symptoms during the day (if daytime wetting is also present, see combined section)
- A child may sleep deeply and be unaware of accidents
- Occasional embarrassment or reluctance to participate in sleepovers

Differentiation from Other Urinary Issues

- Children with **UTIs or diabetes** may wet the bed along with other symptoms like pain, excessive thirst, or foul-smelling urine
- If bedwetting is accompanied by **daytime incontinence**, further evaluation is needed

Seek Immediate Medical Treatment

- Bedwetting begins after 6+ months of dry nights (secondary enuresis)
- Accompanied by pain during urination, frequent urination, or fever
- If the child complains of urgency or accidents during the day as well
- Family history of kidney or bladder problems
- Signs of stress, anxiety, or behavioral changes

- Child is over age 7 and wetting is causing social or emotional distress

Possible Medical Conditions to Consider:

- Urinary tract infection
- Constipation causing bladder pressure
- Sleep disorders (including obstructive sleep apnea)
- Type 1 diabetes (if accompanied by excessive thirst and urination)
- Neurological conditions (rare, but considered if daytime symptoms or developmental delays exist)

Comfort Care and Natural Remedies for Bedwetting:

1. Bladder Training During the Day

Rationale:

Gradually increasing the time between bathroom visits during the day can help expand bladder capacity and awareness of fullness cues.

Instructions:

a. Encourage your child to delay urination for a few minutes when the urge arises, gradually extending the time as tolerated.
b. Remind them to void at regular intervals rather than waiting until the last moment.
c. Keep a log to track progress and make it a positive experience.

Precaution:

- Avoid excessive holding that causes discomfort or accidents.
- Do not use this technique in children with daytime wetting unless directed by a provider.

2. Herbal Nervine Support

Rationale:

Calming herbs like chamomile, lemon balm, or skullcap can support restful sleep and reduce anxiety or nervous tension that may contribute to deep, unresponsive sleep.

Instructions:

a. For children over age 1, steep 1 tsp of dried herb (or a blend) in 1 cup hot water.
b. Let steep 5–10 minutes, then cool completely.
c. Offer in small sips before bedtime, up to ½ cup.
d. Alternatively, use pediatric tincture drops under supervision or guidance of a trained provider.

Precaution:

- Do not use herbal teas in infants under 12 months.
- Always check dosing if using a tincture or combination formula.

3. Limit Fluids After Dinner

Rationale:

Reducing fluid intake in the evening lowers nighttime urine production and decreases the chance of bedwetting episodes.

Instructions:

a. Encourage generous hydration earlier in the day.
b. Reduce fluid intake 1 to 2 hours before bedtime.
c. Offer only small sips if the child requests a drink close to bedtime.

Precaution:

- Ensure your child still receives enough daily fluid to prevent constipation or dehydration.
- Never restrict fluids excessively.

4. Scheduled Nighttime Bathroom Trips

Rationale:

Waking a child once during the night to use the toilet can reinforce bladder awareness and reduce nighttime accidents.

Instructions:

a. Have the child urinate immediately before bedtime.
b. Gently wake them once during the night, around the time accidents typically occur.
c. Be consistent for a few weeks to help build routine.

Precaution:

- Do not wake the child multiple times per night, as sleep disruption may affect mood or cognition.
- Use only short-term unless guided by a provider.

5. Use of Moisture Alarms (For Older Children)

Rationale:

Moisture alarms detect the first sign of urine and alert the child to wake, helping condition a quicker response to bladder fullness during sleep.

Instructions:

a. Attach the moisture sensor to your child's undergarments per device instructions.
b. Place the alarm unit near the bed or on the child's shoulder.
c. Use nightly for at least 4 to 8 weeks for optimal results.
d. Offer positive reinforcement without punishment.

Precaution:

- Best used in children over age 6 who are motivated and ready to participate.
- Do not use without adult supervision.
- May cause sleep disturbance in the short term.

Supportive Practices

- Avoid shame or punishment—bedwetting is not your child's fault.
- Use mattress protectors and absorbent bedding for comfort and ease of cleaning.
- Praise dry nights and effort with gentle encouragement.
- Offer a sticker chart or small rewards to support progress.
- Address emotional stress, anxiety, or school-related concerns that may be contributing.

Urinary Retention and Daytime Wetting

Urinary retention refers to the inability or difficulty in fully emptying the bladder, while **daytime wetting (diurnal enuresis)** involves involuntary leakage of urine during waking hours. These conditions may occur separately or together and can stem from behavioral, emotional, structural, or neurological causes.

Signs and Symptoms of urinary retention and daytime wetting:

- Infrequent urination despite adequate fluid intake
- Difficulty starting the urine stream or weak strea
- Dribbling or damp underwear during the day
- Holding behaviors (crossed legs, squatting, dancing, holding genitals)
- Urgency or rushing to the toilet but not making it in time
- History of constipation
- Sudden onset of accidents after previous dryness
- Complaints of lower abdominal discomfort or fullness

Differentiation from Other Urinary Issues:

- **UTIs** may involve wetting but usually include burning, fever, and foul-smelling urine
- **Primary enuresis** refers only to nighttime bedwetting without daytime symptoms
- **Constipation** is often an underlying or aggravating factor in retention and wetting

Seek Immediate Medical Treatment

- Persistent daytime wetting in a child over age 5
- Pain or difficulty when trying to urinate
- Signs of urinary retention or bladder fullness without successful urination

- Sudden change in bathroom habits with behavioral shifts
- Child complains of discomfort, pressure, or abdominal pain
- History of UTIs or suspected spinal or neurological issues

Comfort Care and Natural Strategies:

1. Address Underlying Constipation

Rationale:

Constipation can cause stool to press against the bladder, affecting its function and contributing to both daytime wetting and retention. Managing bowel health helps relieve bladder pressure and improves control.

Instructions:

a. Increase dietary fiber using fruits, vegetables, and whole grains.
b. Encourage hydration with water and gentle teas like marshmallow root.
c. For children over 1 year, offer 1–2 oz of diluted prune or pear juice daily.
d. Consider magnesium citrate in pediatric formulations under medical supervision if bowel movements remain infrequent.

Precaution:

- Always consult a pediatrician before using magnesium or herbal teas in young children.
- Avoid overuse of juice to prevent diarrhea.

2. Bladder Training Exercises

Rationale:

Bladder training helps improve awareness of urinary signals, strengthens control, and promotes complete voiding.

Instructions:

a. Encourage the child to hold their urine for 5–10 minutes when safe to do so, gradually increasing the interval.
b. Practice "double voiding" by having them urinate, wait one minute, and attempt to urinate again.
c. Reinforce a calm and relaxed posture on the toilet to fully empty the bladder.

Precaution:

- Do not force holding if it causes discomfort.
- Avoid bladder training during active urinary tract infections.

3. Emotional and Behavioral Support

Rationale:

Emotional stress, anxiety, or traumatic experiences can influence bladder control. Creating a safe, calm environment supports healing and trust.

Instructions:

a. Offer consistent emotional validation and reassure your child that accidents are not their fault.
b. Avoid blame or punishment.
c. Incorporate calming routines such as mindfulness, nature walks, creative play, or journaling.
d. Seek counseling if needed for trauma or significant behavioral concerns.

Precaution:

- If anxiety or trauma is suspected, consult a pediatric mental health provider.
- Maintain privacy and dignity in discussions about toileting.

4. Encourage Regular Bathroom Breaks

Rationale:

Children often delay urination during play or school, leading to overstretched bladders and accidents. Scheduled voiding supports bladder health.

Instructions:

a. Create a schedule for bathroom breaks every 2–3 hours, regardless of urge.
b. Use gentle reminders or a visual chart to help maintain consistency.
c. Offer praise for participation without pressure.

Precaution:

- Do not scold or rush the child during bathroom breaks.
- Adjust the schedule if it causes distress or resistance.

5. Ensure Comfortable Bathroom Access

Rationale:

Avoidance of unpleasant or restrictive restroom environments can contribute to holding behaviors and retention.

Instructions:

a. Speak with teachers and caregivers about allowing free bathroom access.
b. At home, provide a clean, quiet, and well-lit space for toileting.
c. Use a footstool to support the child's feet and promote a relaxed squatting posture if needed.

Precaution:

- If school policies limit access, request a note from the pediatrician.
- Address any sensory concerns or fears about public toilets.

Frequent Urination (Pollakiuria)

Frequent urination, or pollakiuria, refers to an increased need to urinate more often than usual, typically without an increase in urine volume. In children, this is often benign and temporary, but it may also signal underlying issues if persistent.

Causes

- Stress or anxiety (common trigger in school-aged children)
- Recent changes in routine (e.g., starting school, family transitions)
- Increased fluid intake
- Constipation causing pressure on the bladder
- Bladder overactivity
- Habitual or learned behaviors
- Less commonly, urinary tract infection (UTI) or diabetes mellitus

Signs and Symptoms:

- Urinating every 10–30 minutes or more than 8 times during the day
- Small amounts of urine each time
- No pain or burning (if pain is present, consider UTI or irritation)
- No fever or other signs of illness
- Typically no wetting accidents at night
- May coincide with stress, anxiety, or a recent life change (school, new sibling, etc.)

Differentiation from Other Urinary Issues:

- **UTIs** are usually accompanied by pain, odor, or fever
- **Diabetes** may cause frequent urination along with thirst, weight loss, or fatigue

- **Constipation** can cause bladder pressure and mimic urinary urgency.

Seek Immediate Medical Treatment

- Frequent urination persists beyond 1–2 weeks
- Accompanied by pain, burning, fever, blood in urine, or bedwetting
- Child has excessive thirst, weight loss, or lethargy (rule out diabetes)
- Child is anxious, withdrawn, or displaying other emotional signs
- Any concerns about the sudden onset or disruption of daily life

Comfort Care and Natural Strategies:

1. Address Underlying Stress or Anxiety

Rationale:

Emotional stress is one of the most common causes of benign frequent urination in children. Calming the nervous system can reduce overactive bladder signaling.

Instructions:

a. Create a predictable routine with a calm bedtime wind-down.
b. Engage the child in regular calming activities such as reading, art, nature walks, or play.
c. Consider gentle herbal support such as chamomile or lemon balm tea for children over 1 year old.
d. Encourage open communication and offer reassurance without focusing excessively on the issue.

Precaution:

- Always consult a pediatrician before introducing herbal remedies.
- Discontinue any herbal product if an allergic reaction or intolerance is observed.

2. Bladder Training (if appropriate)

Rationale:

Bladder training helps restore awareness and control by teaching the child to void on a consistent schedule and resist unnecessary urges.

Instructions:

a. Encourage the child to void every 2–3 hours during the day, whether they feel the urge or not.
b. If safe and without discomfort, ask the child to delay urination briefly when the urge arises, gradually increasing time.
c. Track voiding intervals using a sticker chart to reinforce progress.

Precaution:

- Do not force holding if the child experiences pain or significant urgency.
- Avoid bladder training in children with a history of urinary tract infections or known bladder dysfunction without medical supervision.

3. Ensure Regular Bowel Movements

Rationale:

Constipation can place pressure on the bladder and cause urinary frequency or urgency. Managing bowel health can help reduce symptoms.

Instructions:

a. Encourage a diet high in fiber with fruits, vegetables, and whole grains.
b. Ensure daily hydration.
c. Consider natural supports like prune puree, diluted pear juice, or gentle abdominal massage for infants and toddlers.

Precaution:

- Avoid giving large amounts of juice to infants under 1 year.
- Consult with a provider if constipation persists or worsens.

4. Monitor Fluid Intake

Rationale:

Balancing fluid intake helps prevent both dehydration and excessive bladder stimulation. Some children may overhydrate due to attention or habit.

Instructions:

a. Offer regular fluids during the day, but limit excess drinking in the evening.
b. Avoid caffeinated or citrus-based beverages, which may irritate the bladder.
c. Encourage plain water as the primary drink.

Precaution:

- Avoid fluid restriction to the point of dehydration.
- Speak with a pediatrician if the child seems excessively thirsty or constantly requests water.

5. Reassure the Child

Rationale:

Frequent urination may resolve on its own with reassurance and reduced anxiety around bathroom habits.

Instructions:

a. Explain to your child that this is a common and often temporary experience.
b. Avoid drawing attention or expressing frustration about bathroom frequency.
c. Create a calm environment and normalize bathroom use without pressure.

Precaution:

- Monitor for signs of escalating anxiety or obsessive behaviors.
- Seek help if the child becomes distressed, embarrassed, or socially withdrawn due to the condition.

Constipation-Related Urinary Symptoms

Constipation occurs when a child has infrequent, hard, or painful bowel movements. Due to the close anatomical relationship between the rectum and bladder, retained stool can press against the bladder, leading to urinary symptoms such as urgency, frequency, wetting, or incomplete bladder emptying.

Signs and Symptoms:

- Infrequent bowel movements (less than 3 per week)
- Large, hard, or painful stools
- Stool withholding behaviors (crossed legs, clenching, hiding)
- Abdominal bloating or discomfort
- Daytime wetting or accidents
- Urinary frequency or urgency without infection
- Recurrent urinary tract infections (especially in girls)

Differentiation from Other Urinary Issues:

- If urinary symptoms improve after a bowel movement, constipation is a likely contributor
- Children with **normal urine tests but persistent wetting** should be assessed for constipation
- Constipation-related urinary symptoms often coexist with encopresis (soiling)

Seek Immediate Medical Treatment

- The child has not had a bowel movement in several days and is showing signs of discomfort
- Persistent urinary symptoms with no clear urinary cause
- History of recurrent UTIs or incomplete bladder emptying
- Stool withholding with abdominal distention or vomiting
- Soiling accidents in toilet-trained children

For natural remedies, see chapter 6 under "constipation."

CHAPTER 08

SKIN HEALTH

This section is for educational purposes only. The remedies listed are intended to support comfort and wellness and should not be used as a substitute for professional medical advice. Always consult your child's healthcare provider for diagnosis and treatment.

Diaper Rash (Irritant Diaper Dermatitis)

Diaper rash is inflammation of the skin in the diaper area, usually caused by prolonged moisture, friction, or contact with urine and stool. It is extremely common in infants and young toddlers.

Causes:

- Prolonged exposure to wet or soiled diapers
- Friction from diaper rubbing
- Sensitivity to wipes, soaps, or detergents
- Introduction of new foods (changing stool consistency)
- Antibiotic use (may promote yeast overgrowth)

Signs and Symptoms:

- Redness or raw patches on the buttocks, genitals, or upper thighs
- Irritability or crying during diaper changes
- Peeling, swelling, or open skin in more severe cases
- In some cases, small red spots or satellite lesions indicating yeast involvement

Seek Immediate Medical Attention:

- Rash spreads beyond diaper area or oozes pus
- Accompanied by fever or blisters
- Signs of secondary infection (yellow crusting, rapid worsening)
- Rash persists beyond 72 hours despite home care

Natural Remedies and Comfort Measures for Diaper Rash

1. *Fresh Aloe or Aloe Vera Gel*

Rationale:

Aloe vera has soothing, anti-inflammatory, and antimicrobial properties that can calm irritated skin and support healing.

Instructions:

a. Use pure, food-grade aloe vera gel (no added alcohol, fragrances, or dyes).
b. Apply a thin layer to clean, dry skin after each diaper change.
c. Allow to air dry before replacing diaper.

Precaution:

- Do not use on broken skin or if the child shows signs of an aloe allergy.

2. *Apple Cider Vinegar Rinse*

Rationale:

ACV helps balance the skin's pH and discourage yeast or bacterial overgrowth.

Instructions:

a. Mix 1 tablespoon of raw, unfiltered apple cider vinegar into 1 cup of warm water.
b. Gently dab onto affected area using a soft cloth or cotton pad after cleaning.
c. Let the area fully dry before applying a barrier cream.

Precaution:

- Do not use on cracked or open skin. Discontinue use if irritation occurs.

3. Bentonite Clay Paste

Rationale:

Bentonite clay helps absorb moisture and toxins while forming a gentle barrier.

Instructions:

a. Mix bentonite clay with a small amount of breast milk or distilled water to form a paste.
b. Apply a thin layer to the rash.
c. Let sit 5–10 minutes or allow to dry before re-diapering.
d. Use up to 2 times daily during flare-ups.

Precaution:

- Do not apply to open or bleeding skin.

4. Breast Milk Application

Rationale:

Breast milk contains natural antibodies and enzymes that soothe and protect irritated skin.

Instructions:

a. Express a few drops of breast milk onto clean fingers.
b. Gently apply to the rash and allow it to air dry.
c. Reapply after each diaper change.

Precaution:

- Not for use on broken or oozing skin.

5. Breast Milk & Bentonite Clay Combo Paste

Rationale:

Combining soothing breast milk with absorbent bentonite clay creates a healing, moisture-wicking layer.

Instructions:

a. Mix a few drops of breast milk into bentonite clay until a spreadable paste forms.
b. Apply gently to the affected area.
c. Allow to air dry fully before diapering.

Precaution:

- Do not apply to cracked or infected skin. Monitor closely for signs of sensitivity.

6. Calendula or Zinc-Based Cream

Rationale:

Calendula reduces inflammation and promotes healing, while zinc oxide provides a protective barrier.

Instructions:

a. Choose a fragrance-free calendula or zinc-based cream.
b. Apply a thin, even layer to clean, dry skin with each diaper change.
c. Use regularly during flare-ups.

Precaution:

- Avoid steroid-containing creams unless prescribed.

7. Chamomile Compress

Rationale:

Chamomile has natural anti-inflammatory and skin-soothing properties.

Instructions:

a. Brew a weak chamomile tea using 1 tea bag in 1 cup hot water.
b. Allow to cool to lukewarm.

c. Soak a clean cloth or cotton pad and gently compress on the rash for 5–10 minutes.
d. Pat dry and apply a protective balm afterward.

Precaution:

- Do not use on children allergic to ragweed or related herbs.

8. Coconut Oil or Tallow Balm

Rationale:

These natural fats soothe inflammation and form a mild moisture barrier on sensitive skin.

Instructions:

a. Use organic virgin coconut oil or grass-fed tallow balm.
b. Apply a thin layer to the diaper area after cleansing and drying.
c. Reapply after each diaper change.

Precaution:

- Discontinue if rash worsens or spreads.

9. Cornstarch

Rationale:

Helps keep the area dry by absorbing moisture and reducing friction.

Instructions:

a. Lightly sprinkle a small amount of cornstarch onto clean, dry skin.
b. Apply before diapering during hot or humid conditions.
c. Use only short-term to avoid buildup.

Precaution:

- Avoid if rash appears fungal, as cornstarch may worsen yeast overgrowth.

10. Emu Oil

Rationale:

Emu oil is deeply moisturizing and has anti-inflammatory benefits suitable for sensitive infant skin.

Instructions:

a. Use pure, high-quality emu oil.
b. Gently massage a small amount onto clean, dry skin.
c. Use 1–2 times daily as needed.

Precaution:

- Do not apply to broken skin. Always patch test first.

11. Frequent Diaper Changes

Rationale:

Frequent changing prevents prolonged exposure to moisture and irritants.

Instructions:

a. Check the diaper every 1–2 hours.
b. Change immediately after bowel movements.
c. Gently pat dry (do not rub).
d. Allow diaper-free time to air out the skin.

Precaution:

- Avoid using alcohol-based wipes. Use water or fragrance-free cloth wipes.

12. Manuka Honey Balm

Rationale:

Manuka honey has antimicrobial and wound-healing properties, helping soothe and protect inflamed skin.

Instructions:

a. Use a pediatric-formulated balm containing medical-grade Manuka honey.
b. Apply a thin layer to affected area after cleaning.
c. Reapply as needed, especially overnight.

Precaution:

- Not for infants under 1 year. Do not use if allergic to honey or bee products.

13. Oatmeal or Baking Soda Bath

Rationale:

Calms inflammation and soothes widespread irritation.

Instructions:

a. Add ¼ cup colloidal oatmeal or 2 tbsp baking soda to a lukewarm bath.
b. Soak baby for 10–15 minutes.
c. Pat dry and apply a protective balm.

Precaution:

- Never leave baby unattended. Use caution to prevent slipping.

Eczema (Atopic Dermatitis)

Eczema, also known as atopic dermatitis, is a chronic inflammatory skin condition that causes dryness, itching, and irritation. It commonly affects infants and young children and may present in patches on the face, scalp, trunk, and creases of the elbows and knees. Flare-ups can be triggered by allergens, irritants, temperature changes, or stress.

Causes:

- Genetic predisposition (family history of eczema, asthma, or allergies)
- Environmental allergens (dust, pollen, pet dander)
- Skin irritants (soaps, detergents, fragrances)
- Food sensitivities (e.g., dairy, eggs, wheat)
- Dry air or temperature changes
- Stress or immune imbalance

Signs & Symptoms:

In Infants & Toddlers:

- Dry, red, scaly patches on cheeks, scalp, or trunk
- Itching that leads to fussiness or disturbed sleep
- Oozing or crusting during flare-ups
- Skin thickening with repeated scratching
- Older Children May Experience:
- Itchy, inflamed skin in the elbows, knees, neck, or wrists
- Skin discoloration or rough texture in affected areas
- Flare-ups worsened by heat, sweat, or stress
- Scratching that leads to open sores or infections

Seek Immediate Medical Attention:

- Signs of skin infection: yellow crusting, pus, warmth, swelling
- Rapid worsening despite home care

- Oozing or bleeding from scratching
- Associated fever or lymph node swelling
- Rash that interferes with sleep, eating, or hydration

Natural Remedies and Comfort Care for Eczema

1. Aloe Vera Gel

Rationale:

Aloe vera is soothing, cooling, and anti-inflammatory. It helps calm itching and supports the healing of inflamed skin.

Instructions:

a. Use only pure, alcohol-free aloe vera gel.
b. Apply a thin layer to clean, dry areas 1–2 times per day.
c. Allow it to dry before applying a moisturizer.

Precaution:

- Do not use on open or oozing skin.
- Perform a patch test before full application.

2. Apple Cider Vinegar Dilution (Soothing Rinse)

Rationale:

Helps restore natural skin pH and may reduce bacteria that aggravate eczema.

Instructions:

a. Dilute 1 tablespoon of raw apple cider vinegar in 1 cup of warm water.
b. Use a clean cloth to gently dab onto affected areas.
c. Rinse with water after a few minutes, then moisturize.

Precaution:

- Do not use on cracked or broken skin.

- Discontinue use if irritation worsens.

3. Calendula or Chamomile Cream

Rationale:

Both herbs reduce inflammation and soothe irritated skin. Calendula promotes healing, and chamomile calms itching.

Instructions:

a. Choose an unscented, alcohol-free herbal cream.
b. Apply 1–3 times daily on clean skin.
c. May be used under a barrier balm or emollient.

Precaution:

- Avoid if the child has ragweed or plant allergies (chamomile is in the same family).
- Discontinue if redness or worsening occurs.

4. Chamomile Compress

Rationale:

Chamomile is calming and helps relieve itching during flare-ups.

Instructions:

a. Brew 1 chamomile tea bag in 1 cup of hot water.
b. Cool to lukewarm and soak a clean cloth in the tea.
c. Apply to affected areas for 10 minutes, then pat dry.

Precaution:

- Not recommended for children with known ragweed allergies.
- Use only when cooled to avoid burns.

5. Emu Oil

Rationale:

Emu oil deeply moisturizes and reduces inflammation without clogging pores. It is especially helpful for dry, thickened patches.

Instructions:

a. Apply a few drops of pure emu oil to clean, damp skin.
b. Gently massage into affected areas 1–2 times daily.
c. Use consistently for best results.

Precaution:

- Perform a patch test before widespread use.
- Do not apply to broken skin.

6. Herbal Tea for Immune and Skin Support (Age 2+)

Rationale:

Herbs like red clover, nettle, and calendula support detoxification and promote healthy skin from within.

Instructions:

a. Steep 1 tsp dried herbs in 1 cup hot water.
b. Cool completely before offering to child.
c. Serve 1–2 tablespoons at a time, once or twice daily.
d. Can be mixed into juice or smoothies.

Precaution:

- Not for children under 2 year.
- Monitor for allergic reaction.

7. Identify and Eliminate Triggers

Rationale:

Preventing exposure to environmental or dietary irritants reduces flare-up frequency.

Instructions:

a. Use quality, fragrance-free laundry detergent and avoid dryer sheets.
b. Dress child in soft, breathable cotton (organice if possible) fabrics.
c. Keep nails trimmed to prevent skin injury from scratching.
d. Discuss potential food triggers with a provider before starting an elimination diet.

Precaution:

- Never eliminate major food groups without professional guidance.
- Avoid restrictive diets unless advised by a pediatric provider.

8. Manuka Honey Balm

Rationale:

Medical-grade Manuka honey has antimicrobial and healing properties and helps reduce inflammation.

Instructions:

a. Use a pediatric-formulated balm or salve with certified Manuka honey.
b. Apply a thin layer to clean skin once or twice daily.
c. Cover lightly with cotton if needed.

Precaution:

- Not for infants under 1 year due to botulism risk.

- Avoid if child has bee or honey allergies.

9. Natural Skin Moisturizers (Tallow, Shea Butter, Coconut Oil)

Rationale:

Natural oils and butters hydrate deeply and protect the skin barrier to reduce eczema symptoms.

Instructions:

a. After bathing, pat skin dry and apply a generous layer to damp skin.
b. Use 1–2 times daily, especially during dry weather.
c. Continue daily use even during periods of improvement.

Precaution:

- Avoid scented or mixed-product versions.
- Perform a patch test before first use.

10. Oatmeal Bath

Rationale:

Colloidal oatmeal contains anti-inflammatory and antioxidant compounds that calm itchiness and reduce redness.

Instructions:

a. Blend ¼ cup oats into a fine powder.
b. Add to lukewarm bathwater and soak for 10–15 minutes.
c. Pat skin dry and moisturize immediately afterward.

Precaution:

- Always supervise child during bath.
- Ensure water is lukewarm, not hot.

11. Wet Wrap Therapy

Rationale:

Wet wrap therapy is highly effective during intense flare-ups by locking in moisture and allowing emollients to absorb deeply. It also reduces itching and promotes faster healing.

Instructions:

a. Bathe the child in lukewarm water for 10–15 minutes and gently pat dry.
b. Apply a thick layer of an **emollient** (such as petroleum jelly, shea butter, tallow balm, or fragrance-free barrier ointments like Aquaphor or Vanicream) to the affected skin.
c. Wrap the area with clean, **damp** cotton cloths or gauze.
d. Cover with a **dry** layer such as pajamas or cotton clothing.
e. Leave wraps on for 1–2 hours or overnight if recommended by a provider.
f. Remove wraps and reapply moisturizer.

Precaution:

- Do not use over broken or infected skin.
- Always use fresh, clean wraps.
- Monitor the child to ensure warmth and comfort.

Natural Skin Moisturizers

Moisturizing the skin is vital to pediatric skin health, particularly after illness, skin irritation, or exposure to the elements. Children's skin is more delicate than adult skin and loses moisture more easily, which can lead to dryness, cracking, or a compromised skin barrier. Using natural oils and butters helps lock in hydration, protect against environmental damage, and support the body's natural healing processes.

The following natural moisturizers can be used alone or blended with others to soothe dry, sensitive, or healing skin. Most are safe for daily use, though patch testing is recommended before first use in sensitive children.

- **Beef Tallow (Grass-Fed):**

  Rich in vitamins A, D, E, and K, beef tallow is biologically compatible with human skin. It nourishes deeply, mimics natural sebum, and helps repair damaged or dry skin. Ideal for sensitive or eczema-prone areas.

- **Olive Oil (Extra Virgin):**

  This antioxidant-rich oil moisturizes and softens the skin while protecting against oxidative damage. It is gentle enough for infants and can be used as a massage oil or daily moisturizer.

- **Coconut Oil (Virgin, Cold-Pressed):**

  Naturally antimicrobial and anti-inflammatory, coconut oil creates a light protective layer that helps retain moisture and soothe dry or irritated patches.

- **Emu Oil:**

  Penetrates deeply into the skin and carries nutrients below the surface. It is rich in omega fatty acids and is especially beneficial for inflamed or recovering skin, including after burns or rashes.

- **Vitamin E Oil:**

A powerful antioxidant that supports skin regeneration and minimizes scarring. Use sparingly on healing skin, especially after wounds or stretch marks.

- **Sea Moss Gel:**

  High in minerals and humectant properties, sea moss gel hydrates while supporting skin elasticity and barrier repair. It is especially beneficial for dry, rough skin.

- **Shea Butter (Raw, Unrefined):**

  Shea butter contains natural healing fats and is effective at sealing in moisture and protecting against environmental irritants. It works well for chapped skin, windburn, or dry patches.

- **Breast Milk (Topical Use):**

  Breast milk contains natural antibodies, enzymes, and fats that moisturize, reducing inflammation and infection risk. It can be applied to irritation, rash, or dryness in young infants.

- **Calendula Oil:**

  Made by infusing calendula flowers in a carrier oil, this gentle anti-inflammatory oil calms sensitive, rashy, or post-burn skin. It is particularly useful for infants and toddlers with reactive skin.

- **Jojoba Oil:**

  Jojoba is a liquid wax closely resembling the skin's natural oils. It is quickly absorbed and does not clog pores, making it an excellent daily moisturizer for all ages.

- **Castor Oil:**

  Thicker than other oils, castor oil is deeply emollient and works well on cracked heels, lips, or elbows. It can be combined with lighter oils like jojoba or olive oil to make it easier to apply.

- **Avocado Oil:**

  Rich in essential fatty acids, avocado oil deeply nourishes dry or flaking skin and supports skin cell turnover. It is suitable for children with dry or sun-exposed skin.

- **Aloe Vera Gel (Pure):**

  Cooling and hydrating, aloe vera gel is ideal for mild burns, sunburns, or skin needing moisture without greasiness. Always use pure, food-grade aloe without additives.

Heat Rash (Prickly Heat / Miliaria)

Heat rash occurs when sweat becomes trapped in blocked pores, causing inflammation and skin irritation. It is common in babies and young children due to their underdeveloped sweat glands and tendency to overheat.

Causes:

- Hot, humid weather
- Overdressing or tightly swaddled infants
- Prolonged sweating or fever
- Occlusive lotions or synthetic clothing
- Friction in skin folds or tight areas

Signs and Symptoms:

- Small red or pink bumps, often clustered
- Rash appears on neck, back, chest, or in skin folds
- Mild itching, discomfort, or fussiness in babies
- Clear fluid-filled bumps in some cases (miliaria crystallina)

Differentiation from Other Skin Conditions:

- Unlike contact dermatitis, heat rash is not caused by an external allergen or irritant.
- Heat rash is often mistaken for baby acne or allergic rash but lacks pus, widespread inflammation, or a spreading pattern.
- It does not typically ooze, crust, or cause systemic symptoms like fever unless secondary infection occurs.

Seek Immediate Medical Attention:

- Rash spreads rapidly or becomes painful
- Presence of pus, crusting, or signs of infection
- Accompanied by fever or lethargy

- Rash persists longer than 3–5 days without improvement

Natural Remedies and Comfort Care for Heat Rash

1. *Aloe Vera Gel*

Rationale:

Aloe vera is soothing, cooling, and anti-inflammatory. It helps calm itching and supports healing of inflamed skin.

Instructions:

a. Use only pure, alcohol-free aloe vera gel.
b. Apply a thin layer to clean, dry areas 1–2 times per day.
c. Allow it to dry before applying a moisturizer.

Precaution:

- Do not use on open or oozing skin.
- Perform a patch test before full application.

2. *Apple Cider Vinegar Dilution (Soothing Rinse)*

Rationale:

Helps restore natural skin pH and may reduce bacteria that aggravate eczema.

Instructions:

a. Dilute 1 tablespoon of raw apple cider vinegar in 1 cup of warm water.
b. Use a clean cloth to gently dab onto affected areas.
c. Rinse with water after a few minutes, then moisturize.

Precaution:

- Do not use on cracked or broken skin.
- Discontinue use if irritation worsens.

3. Calendula or Chamomile Cream

Rationale:

Both herbs reduce inflammation and soothe irritated skin. Calendula promotes healing, and chamomile calms itching.

Instructions:

a. Choose an unscented, alcohol-free herbal cream.
b. Apply 1–3 times daily on clean skin.
c. May be used under a barrier balm or emollient.

Precaution:

- Avoid if the child has ragweed or plant allergies (chamomile is in the same family).
- Discontinue if redness or worsening occurs.

4. Chamomile Compress

Rationale:

Chamomile is calming and helps relieve itching during flare-ups.

Instructions:

a. Brew 1 chamomile tea bag in 1 cup of hot water.
b. Cool to lukewarm and soak a clean cloth in the tea.
c. Apply to affected areas for 10 minutes, then pat dry.

Precaution:

- Not recommended for children with known ragweed allergies.
- Use only when cooled to avoid burns.

5. Emu Oil

Rationale:

Emu oil deeply moisturizes and reduces inflammation without clogging pores. It is especially helpful for dry, thickened patches.

Instructions:

a. Apply a few drops of pure emu oil to clean, damp skin.
b. Gently massage into affected areas 1–2 times daily.
c. Use consistently for best results.

Precaution:

- Perform a patch test before widespread use
- Do not apply to broken skin.

6. *Epsom Salt Bath (For Children Over Age 2)*

Rationale:

Epsom salt contains magnesium, which may help reduce inflammation and soothe itching skin.

Instructions:

a. Add ½ cup of Epsom salt to a lukewarm bath.
b. Soak the child for 10–15 minutes.
c. Pat dry gently and apply a moisturizer immediately after.

Precaution:

- Not for children under 2 years of age.
- Always supervise during baths to prevent slipping.

7. *Evening Primrose Oil (Topical Only)*

Rationale:

Evening primrose oil is rich in gamma-linolenic acid, which may improve skin hydration and reduce inflammation.

Instructions:

a. Use only cold-pressed, hexane-free evening primrose oil.
b. Apply a small amount to clean, dry patches once or twice daily.

c. Gently massage into skin and follow with a moisturizer.

Precaution:

- For external use only. Do not give orally.
- Perform a patch test before widespread use.

8. Herbal Tea for Immune and Skin Support (Age 1+)

Rationale:

Herbs like red clover, nettle, and calendula support detoxification and promote healthy skin from within.

Instructions:

a. Steep 1 tsp dried herbs in 1 cup hot water.
b. Cool completely before offering to child.
c. Serve 1–2 tablespoons at a time, once or twice daily.
d. Can be mixed into juice or smoothies.

Precaution:

- Not for children under 1 year.
- Monitor for allergic reaction.

9. Identify and Eliminate Triggers

Rationale:

Preventing exposure to environmental or dietary irritants reduces flare-up frequency.

Instructions:

a. Use fragrance-free laundry detergent and avoid dryer sheets.
b. Dress child in soft, breathable cotton fabrics.
c. Keep nails trimmed to prevent skin injury from scratching.

d. Discuss potential food triggers with a provider before starting an elimination diet.

Precaution:

- Never eliminate major food groups without professional guidance.
- Avoid restrictive diets unless advised by a pediatric provider.

10. Manuka Honey Balm

Rationale:

Medical-grade Manuka honey has antimicrobial and healing properties and helps reduce inflammation.

Instructions:

a. Use a pediatric-formulated balm or salve with certified Manuka honey.
b. Apply a thin layer to clean skin once or twice daily.
c. Cover lightly with cotton if needed.

Precaution:

- Not for infants under 1 year due to botulism risk.
- Avoid if child has bee or honey allergies.

11. Natural Skin Moisturizers (Tallow, Shea Butter, Coconut Oil)

Rationale:

Natural oils and butters hydrate deeply and protect the skin barrier to reduce eczema symptoms.

Instructions:

a. After bathing, pat skin dry and apply a generous layer to damp skin.

b. Use 1–2 times daily, especially during dry weather.
c. Continue daily use even during periods of improvement.

Precaution:

- Avoid scented or mixed-product versions.
- Perform a patch test before first use.

12. Oatmeal Bath

Rationale:

Colloidal oatmeal contains anti-inflammatory and antioxidant compounds that calm itchiness and reduce redness.

Instructions:

a. Blend ¼ cup oats into a fine powder.
b. Add to lukewarm bathwater and soak for 10–15 minutes.
c. Pat skin dry and moisturize immediately afterward.

Precaution:

- Always supervise child during bath.
- Ensure water is lukewarm, not hot.

13. Sunflower Oil

Rationale:

Sunflower oil is rich in linoleic acid, which helps restore the skin barrier and reduce inflammation.

Instructions:

a. Choose cold-pressed, organic sunflower oil.
b. Apply to damp skin after bathing.
c. Use once or twice daily to help maintain moisture.

Precaution:

- Do not use if allergic to sunflower seeds.

- Perform a patch test before use.

14. Wet Wrap Therapy

Rationale:

Wet wrap therapy is highly effective during intense flare-ups by locking in moisture and allowing emollients to absorb deeply. It also reduces itching and promotes faster healing.

Instructions:

a. Bathe the child in lukewarm water for 10–15 minutes and gently pat dry.
b. Apply a thick layer of an emollient (such as petroleum jelly, shea butter, tallow balm, or fragrance-free barrier ointments like Aquaphor or Vanicream) to the affected skin.
c. Wrap the area with clean, damp cotton cloths or gauze.
d. Cover with a dry layer such as pajamas or cotton clothing.
e. Leave wraps on for 1–2 hours or overnight if recommended by a provider.
f. Remove wraps and reapply moisturizer.

Precaution:

- Do not use over broken or infected skin.
- Always use fresh, clean wraps.
- Monitor the child to ensure warmth and comfort.

Contact Dermatitis

Contact dermatitis is skin inflammation caused by direct exposure to an irritant or allergen. It often appears as a red, itchy rash and may include swelling or blisters. It can affect children of all ages and may occur suddenly after contact with a new substance or with repeated exposure over time.

Causes:

- Soaps, shampoos, or detergents
- Diaper wipes or fragrances
- Certain fabrics (e.g., wool or synthetic fibers)
- Topical antibiotics or skincare products
- Plants (e.g., poison ivy, poison oak)
- Nickel or metal from jewelry, buttons, or zippers

Signs and Symptoms:

- Red, dry, itchy skin
- Rash localized to area of contact (e.g., hands, cheeks, diaper area)
- Swelling, peeling, or blistering in severe cases
- Irritability or scratching, especially in infants and toddlers
- Skin may appear raw or weepy in advanced cases

Differentiation from Other Skin Conditions:

- Unlike eczema, contact dermatitis is localized and linked to a specific exposure.
- Diaper rash often overlaps but may improve with barrier creams and better hygiene, while contact dermatitis may persist until the irritant is removed.
- Unlike impetigo or fungal infections, contact dermatitis is not contagious or typically pus-filled.

Seek Immediate Medical Attention:

- Rash is spreading rapidly or blistering
- Associated with facial or eye swelling
- Rash becomes infected (yellow crusting, pus, warmth, fever)
- Symptoms persist beyond 5–7 days despite removing the suspected irritant
- Rash interferes with eating, sleeping, or hydration

Natural Remedies and Comfort Care for Contact Dermatitis

1. Aloe Vera or Calendula Gel

Rationale:

These herbs have natural cooling and anti-inflammatory properties that relieve redness, itching, and irritation.

Instructions:

a. Use pure, alcohol-free aloe vera gel or an unscented calendula cream.
b. Apply a thin layer to clean, dry skin.
c. Repeat 2–3 times daily and allow skin to breathe between applications.

Precaution:

- Avoid products containing fragrance or alcohol.
- Discontinue if rash worsens or signs of allergy occur.

2. Bentonite Clay Paste

Rationale:

Bentonite clay draws out toxins and moisture while creating a soothing, protective layer over irritated skin.

Instructions:

a. Mix 1 tablespoon of bentonite clay with enough distilled water to form a smooth paste.
b. Apply a thin layer to the affected area.
c. Allow to dry for 10–15 minutes, then rinse gently and pat dry.
d. Use once daily during active irritation.

Precaution:

- Do not apply to open or oozing skin.
- Patch test on a small area before full use.

3. Chamomile or Marshmallow Root Compress

Rationale:

These herbs are anti-inflammatory and mucilaginous, helping to calm and protect irritated or inflamed skin.

Instructions:

a. Steep 1–2 teaspoons of dried chamomile or marshmallow root in 1 cup of hot water for 10–15 minutes.
b. Cool the tea completely.
c. Soak a clean cloth in the tea and apply to affected area for 5–10 minutes.
d. Use once or twice daily during flare-ups.

Precaution:

- Ensure the compress is fully cooled before applying.
- Discontinue if redness or rash increases.
- Avoid chamomile if your child has a ragweed allergy.

4. Cold Compress

Rationale:

A cold compress reduces inflammation, swelling, and itching during the early stages of a contact dermatitis flare.

Instructions:

a. Soak a clean washcloth in cool water and wring it out.
b. Place gently on the affected skin for 5–10 minutes.
c. Repeat 2–3 times per day as needed for relief.

Precaution:

- Do not apply ice directly to the skin.
- Stop use if child becomes chilled or uncomfortable.

5. Coconut Oil or Emu Oil for Moisture

Rationale:

These natural oils moisturize and protect the skin, helping prevent further irritation and dryness.

Instructions:

a. Apply a light layer to clean, dry skin after washing.
b. Reapply after bathing or diapering (if applicable).
c. Use 1–2 times daily until the skin is healed.

Precaution:

- Do not apply to oozing, broken, or infected skin
- Always patch test before using a new product.

6. Colloidal Silver Spray (for mild skin support)

Rationale:

Colloidal silver has natural antimicrobial properties and may help reduce surface bacteria on intact, irritated skin.

Instructions:

a. Use a high-quality, pediatric-safe colloidal silver spray.
b. Lightly mist over clean, dry skin.
c. Allow to air dry before applying moisturizer.
d. Use once daily only during flare-ups.

Precaution:

- Use only on intact skin (not on broken or weeping rashes).
- Do not use long term without provider guidance.

7. Epsom Salt Bath (Age 2+)

Rationale:

Epsom salt baths help soothe itching and reduce inflammation while promoting skin detoxification.

Instructions:

a. Add ½ cup of Epsom salt to a lukewarm bath.
b. Soak for 10–15 minutes under adult supervision.
c. Pat skin dry and apply a protective moisturizer.

Precaution:

- Not for use on broken skin or in children under 2.
- Avoid if rash worsens after use.

8. Evening Primrose Oil (Topical Use Only)

Rationale:

Evening primrose oil is high in gamma-linolenic acid, which supports skin hydration and reduces eczema-like inflammation.

Instructions:

a. Use a pure, cold-pressed evening primrose oil product.
b. Apply a few drops to clean, dry skin and massage gently.
c. Use once daily during active irritation.

Precaution:

- For external use only.
- Avoid if the child has known sensitivity to nightshades or similar plants.

9. Identify and Remove the Irritant

Rationale:
The most important step in managing contact dermatitis is eliminating the cause of irritation to promote healing and prevent recurrence.

Instructions:

- Gently rinse the skin with cool or lukewarm water—avoid using soaps.
- Stop using suspected products (e.g., wipes, soaps, lotions, clothing dyes).
- Replace with hypoallergenic, fragrance-free alternatives.

Precaution:

- Do not scrub the skin.
- Avoid reintroducing the suspected irritant until the rash has completely resolved.

10. Oatmeal Paste or Bath

Rationale:

Oatmeal is naturally anti-inflammatory and soothes itching, dryness, and redness.

Instructions:

a. For paste: grind oats into a fine powder and mix with water to form a paste.
b. Apply paste directly to the rash and allow to sit for 10–15 minutes.
c. For bath: add ¼ cup of finely ground oats to a lukewarm bath and soak for 10–15 minutes.
d. Pat skin dry and moisturize immediately.

Precaution:

- Always supervise during baths.
- Avoid hot water, which may worsen irritation.

Impetigo

Impetigo is a highly contagious bacterial skin infection, most commonly caused by *Staphylococcus aureus* or *Streptococcus pyogenes*. It typically affects infants and young children and is characterized by honey-colored crusts, blisters, or red sores, often around the mouth, nose, or hands.

Causes:

- Direct contact with an infected person or surface
- Entry of bacteria through cuts, scrapes, or insect bites
- Poor hygiene or scratching eczema lesions
- Overcrowded environments (daycares, schools)

Signs and Symptoms:

- Red sores or blisters that quickly rupture and ooze
- Formation of golden-yellow, crusted patches
- Itchy or mildly painful rash
- Commonly appears on face, hands, or diaper area
- May be localized or spread to other parts of the body

Differentiation from Other Skin Conditions:

- Unlike contact dermatitis or eczema, impetigo produces honey-colored crusts and spreads quickly if not treated.
- Fungal infections like ringworm present with circular scaling, not crusting.
- Unlike molluscum, impetigo is often weepy and acute, not waxy or dome-shaped.

Seek Immediate Medical Attention:

- Rapid spreading of sores or worsening appearance
- Development of fever, swollen lymph nodes, or signs of systemic infection

- Involvement near the eyes or large surface area
- No improvement within 24–48 hours of natural care
- Signs of MRSA (painful boils or deep abscesses)

Natural Remedies and Comfort Care for Impetigo

Note: These remedies are supportive and not a substitute for antibiotic treatment when prescribed.

1. Colloidal Silver Gel or Spray

Rationale:

Colloidal silver has broad-spectrum antimicrobial properties that may help reduce bacterial colonization and soothe inflamed or irritated skin.

Instructions:

a. Gently cleanse the affected area using water and a soft cloth.
b. Spray or apply a thin layer of colloidal silver gel to dry skin.
c. Allow to air dry completely before covering with breathable gauze or a bandage.
d. Repeat 2–3 times per day.

Precaution:

- For external use only.
- Discontinue use if skin becomes discolored or irritated.

2. Keep the Area Clean and Dry

Rationale:

Maintaining proper skin hygiene helps eliminate surface bacteria, remove crusts, and prevent the spread of infection to other body areas or people.

Instructions:

a. Wash the skin gently using lukewarm water and a mild, natural soap.
b. Avoid scrubbing the area. Pat dry with a clean towel.
c. Assign a dedicated towel and washcloth for the infected child.
d. Wash hands thoroughly after any contact with the lesions.

Precaution:

- Do not share towels, linens, or personal items.
- Avoid popping, scratching, or picking at sores.

3. Manuka Honey (or Raw Honey) Application

Rationale:

Manuka honey contains methylglyoxal, a compound with potent antimicrobial activity, particularly effective against Staphylococcus aureus. It also promotes skin healing and reduces inflammation.

Instructions:

a. After cleaning the skin, apply a small amount of raw or medical-grade Manuka honey directly to the area.
b. Cover with sterile gauze, loosely applied to allow airflow.
c. Change the dressing 1–2 times daily.

Precaution:

- Do not apply near the mouth of infants under 1 year.
- For external use only.

4. Support the Immune System Internally

Rationale:

A resilient immune system aids in faster recovery from bacterial infections and may help prevent future outbreaks.

Instructions:

a. Include immune-supportive foods such as garlic, citrus fruits, leafy greens, and bone broth in the child's diet.
b. Offer pediatric-formulated probiotics to support healthy gut flora (See Remedy #11 under Urinary Tract Infection on page 199).
c. Use age-appropriate elderberry syrup as an immune booster (See Remedy #2 under Strep Throat on page 64).

Precaution:

Avoid honey-containing products in infants under 1 year of age. Always consult a pediatric healthcare provider before starting new supplements.

5. Tea Tree Oil Dilution (Age 2+)

Rationale:

Tea tree oil has natural antibacterial effects and may inhibit strains of Staphylococcus when properly diluted and applied topically.

Instructions:

a. Dilute 1 drop of tea tree essential oil into 1 teaspoon of a carrier oil (such as coconut or olive oil).
b. Apply the diluted oil directly to the lesion using a clean cotton swab.
c. Repeat once daily as a spot treatment.

Precaution:

- Do not apply undiluted tea tree oil directly to skin.
- Avoid using near the eyes, mouth, or on broken skin.
- Not safe for children under 2 years of age.

6. Turmeric Paste

Rationale:
Turmeric contains curcumin, a natural anti-inflammatory and antimicrobial compound that supports the healing of minor skin infections.

Instructions:

a. Mix 1 teaspoon of turmeric powder with filtered water or raw honey to create a thick paste.
b. Apply directly to the lesion and leave on for 10–15 minutes.
c. Rinse gently and pat the skin dry. Use once per day.

Precaution:

- May temporarily stain the skin, fabrics, and clothing.
- Not recommended for use on open or actively oozing wounds.

Molluscum Contagiosum

Molluscum contagiosum is a common viral skin infection caused by the poxvirus. It presents as small, dome-shaped, flesh-colored or pink bumps with a central dimple. It typically affects children between 1 and 10 years of age and spreads easily through skin-to-skin contact or contaminated surfaces.

Causes:

- Direct skin contact with infected individuals
- Sharing towels, clothing, or bath items
- Scratching or rubbing the lesions (autoinoculation)
- Weakened immunity or preexisting skin irritation

Signs and Symptoms:

- Small (2–5 mm), firm, smooth bumps with a central indentation
- May appear singly or in clusters on the face, trunk, arms, or legs
- Usually painless but may become red or itchy
- Occasionally inflamed or red as the body begins to fight the virus
- Most children have 10–20 lesions; outbreaks can last for months

Differentiation from Other Skin Conditions:

- Unlike warts, molluscum has a characteristic central dimple and smoother surface.
- Unlike impetigo, there is no weeping or crusting unless secondarily infected.
- May resemble acne or milia but typically does not involve pus unless irritated or scratched.

Seek Immediate Medical Attention:

- Sudden increase in number or size of lesions
- Signs of secondary bacterial infection (redness, pain, pus, swelling)
- Lesions on or near the eyes or genitals
- Immunocompromised children or those with eczema and worsening symptoms
- Persistent lesions beyond 12 months or significant emotional/social impact

Natural Remedies and Comfort Care for Molluscum Contagiosum

1. Do Not Scratch or Pick Lesions

Rationale:

Scratching spreads the virus to other areas of the skin and increases risk of secondary infection.

Instructions:

a. Keep fingernails short and clean.
b. Use distraction methods or light cotton gloves during sleep if scratching is an issue.
c. Apply a natural itch-relief salve (e.g., calendula or coconut oil) if the skin is dry or irritated.

Precaution:

Avoid squeezing or "popping" lesions to reduce the risk of spreading or scarring.

2. Boost Immune System Naturally

Rationale:

Molluscum resolves when the immune system mounts a response. Supporting immunity may help shorten duration.

Instructions:

a. Provide nutrient-rich foods (bone broth, leafy greens, berries, and garlic).
b. Offer vitamin C-rich options like oranges, strawberries, or elderberry syrup (See #3 under "Strep Throat").
c. Ensure regular outdoor play and restful sleep.

Precaution:

Always supervise use of supplements and avoid honey under 1 year of age.

3. Apple Cider Vinegar Spot Treatment

Rationale:

ACV is mildly antiviral and astringent, helping to dry out lesions over time.

Instructions:

a. Dilute apple cider vinegar 1:1 with filtered water.
b. Apply to a single lesion using a cotton swab once daily.
c. Cover with a small bandage if desired to reduce rubbing or spread.

Precaution:

Do not use on broken skin or near the eyes. May cause stinging—discontinue if irritation worsens.

4. Tea Tree Oil and Iodine Spot Treatment (Age 5+)

Rationale:

Tea tree oil and iodine may have antiviral properties and help shrink the lesions gradually.

Instructions:

a. Mix 1 drop tea tree oil with 1 tsp carrier oil.
b. Dab a small amount onto each lesion using a clean cotton swab.
c. Follow with a trace amount of iodine tincture (if available).
d. Repeat once daily for 2–3 weeks.

Precaution:

Avoid use near eyes or on broken skin. Discontinue if stinging or redness occurs.

5. Colloidal Silver Gel or Spray

Rationale:

Colloidal silver is naturally antimicrobial and may reduce viral load when applied regularly.

Instructions:

a. Apply a small amount of gel or spray directly to clean, dry skin
b. Let air dry. Use 1–2 times daily.
c. May be used in combination with tea tree oil or ACV regimen.

Precaution:

Use only externally. Discontinue if irritation develops.

6. Keep Skin Clean and Covered

Rationale:

Minimizes spread to others and reduces the risk of secondary bacterial infection.

Instructions:

a. Bathe daily with a gentle, fragrance-free cleanser.
b. Cover large or exposed lesions (e.g., during school or sports) with a breathable bandage.
c. Wash clothing, towels, and sheets frequently.

Precaution:

Do not use antibacterial soaps, which may dry and irritate skin.

Ringworm (Tinea Corporis)

Ringworm is a contagious superficial fungal infection that affects the skin, presenting as a round, red, scaly patch with a raised border and clearer center. Despite its name, it is not caused by a worm but by dermatophyte fungi that thrive on warm, moist skin.

Causes:

- Skin contact with an infected person, animal (especially cats), or contaminated surface
- Sharing hats, brushes, towels, clothing, or bedding
- Warm, humid environments and tight clothing
- Weakened immunity or minor skin trauma

Signs and Symptoms:

- Round or oval red lesion with a scaly, raised edge and central clearing
- May appear on arms, trunk, face, or legs
- Lesion slowly expands in size
- Mild to moderate itching
- In some cases, multiple rings may overlap
- Scalp ringworm (tinea capitis) may cause hair loss and scabbing

Differentiation from Other Skin Conditions:

- Unlike eczema, ringworm has a distinct circular border and clear center.
- Unlike impetigo, there is no crusting or pus unless secondarily infected.
- Often confused with nummular eczema but lacks chronic dryness or cracking.
- Molluscum is dome-shaped and smooth—not scaly or ring-like.

Seek Immediate Medical Attention:

- Lesion is near the eyes or spreads rapidly
- Signs of secondary bacterial infection (yellow crusting, swelling, warmth)
- Child is immunocompromised
- Scalp involvement or hair loss (may require oral antifungal treatment)
- No improvement with natural remedies within 7–10 days

Natural Remedies and Comfort Care for Ringworm

Note: Natural remedies may support healing in early or mild cases. If lesions persist or worsen, seek antifungal medication.

1. Apple Cider Vinegar (ACV) Spot Treatment

Rationale:

Apple cider vinegar has antifungal and astringent properties that may help inhibit fungal growth and restore the skin's natural pH.

Instructions:

a. Dilute apple cider vinegar with equal parts water (1:1 ratio)
b. Use a clean cotton swab to dab the solution directly onto the lesion.
c. Allow the area to air dry completely before covering or dressing.
d. Apply 2–3 times daily.

Precaution:

- Do not apply to broken, oozing, or highly sensitive skin.
- Discontinue use if burning, redness, or irritation occurs.

2. Colloidal Silver Gel or Spray

Rationale:

Colloidal silver may help support healing due to its natural antimicrobial and soothing properties, which may reduce skin irritation and inhibit secondary bacterial growth.

Instructions:

a. Clean and dry the area before application.
b. Apply a thin layer of colloidal silver gel or spray directly onto the lesion.
c. Allow to air dry before applying clothing or bandages.
d. Use 2 times daily.

Precaution:

- For external use only.
- Avoid prolonged use beyond 10–14 days unless directed by a healthcare provider.

3. Garlic Paste (Optional for Older Children)

Rationale:

Garlic contains ajoene and allicin—natural compounds with potent antifungal effects that may help suppress the fungal growth causing ringworm.

Instructions:

a. Crush one clove of fresh garlic and mix with a few drops of coconut oil to create a paste.
b. Apply to the lesion and leave on for 5–10 minutes.
c. Rinse gently with warm water and pat dry.
d. Use once daily.

Precaution:

- May cause skin irritation or burning sensation.
- Always perform a patch test before use.

- Not recommended for sensitive skin or children under age 6.

4. Gentian Violet for Ringworm

Rationale:

Gentian violet has antifungal and drying properties that may help inhibit superficial fungal growth and support skin recovery when conventional treatments are unavailable or poorly tolerated.

Instructions:

a. Thoroughly clean and dry the affected skin.
b. Use a cotton swab to apply a thin, even layer directly to the ring-shaped rash.
c. Allow the area to air dry.
d. Use once daily for up to 5 consecutive days.

Precaution:

- Will stain skin temporarily and permanently stain clothing and fabrics.
- Do not use near eyes, mouth, or genital area.
- Avoid prolonged use or applying to large skin areas.
- Discontinue if the rash worsens or spreads and seek medical care.

5. Keep the Area Clean and Dry

Rationale:

Fungi thrive in warm, moist environments. Maintaining dryness and cleanliness helps limit fungal overgrowth and supports the healing process.

Instructions:

a. Wash the affected area once daily using lukewarm water and mild soap.
b. Pat thoroughly dry with a clean towel—avoid rubbing.

c. Change clothing and undergarments daily.
d. Avoid tight, non-breathable fabrics over the lesion.

Precaution:

- Use separate towels for infected areas.
- Wash hands immediately after contact with the rash.

6. Prevent Spread to Others

Rationale:
Ringworm is highly contagious and spreads easily through direct contact and shared items. Preventing transmission protects both the child and others in the home.

Instructions:

a. Avoid scratching or touching the lesion, especially before handwashing.
b. Do not share personal items such as brushes, hats, towels, or clothing.
c. Wash bedding, clothing, and towels in hot water after each use.
d. Keep fingernails trimmed and clean to avoid spreading spores.

Precaution:

- Examine pets for patches of hair loss or lesions and consult a veterinarian if needed.

7. Tea Tree Oil (Age 2+)

Rationale:

Tea tree oil is a widely recognized natural antifungal that may be effective against tinea (ringworm), helping to reduce inflammation and fungal spread.

Instructions:

a. Dilute 1 drop of tea tree oil in 1 teaspoon of carrier oil (e.g., coconut or olive oil).
b. Apply directly to the affected area using a clean cotton swab.
c. Apply twice daily and continue for at least one week after the rash has cleared.

Precaution:

- Never use undiluted essential oils directly on the skin.
- Avoid use near the eyes, mouth, or on the face of young children.
- Not recommended for children under 2 years of age.

Skin Injuries (Cuts, Scrapes, and Abrasions)

Definition:

Skin injuries in children include scrapes (abrasions), shallow cuts (lacerations), and skin tears. These injuries commonly occur from falls, play, or accidents and usually heal well with proper care.

Causes:

- Falls or friction from rough surfaces (playground injuries, bike falls)
- Sharp objects or rough toys
- Nail scratching (especially in infants)
- Accidental cuts during play, sports, or household activity

Signs and Symptoms:

- Redness, bleeding, or raw skin
- Mild swelling or tenderness
- Scab formation as the skin begins to heal
- Itching during later healing stages
- May become infected if not kept clean

Seek Immediate Medical Attention:

- Wounds with deep cuts, exposed fat or muscle, or uncontrolled bleeding
- Objects embedded in the skin
- Wounds that gape open or may need stitches
- Signs of infection (see below)
- Any wound near the eye or genitals
- Wounds that don't improve or show worsening after 48 hours

Stages of Skin Healing

Understanding these phases helps guide appropriate care and reduce long-term scarring.

1. Inflammatory Stage (First 1–3 Days)

Goal: Control bleeding and begin cleaning process

- Skin is red, swollen, and tender.
- The immune system sends white blood cells to prevent infection.

Supportive Care:

a. Gently clean the wound with cool water and mild soap.
b. Apply diluted **colloidal silver spray** or **herbal wash** (chamomile or calendula).
c. Cover with a breathable, clean bandage.
d. Use **raw honey** or **aloe vera** for antibacterial and soothing effects.

2. Proliferative Stage (Days 3–10)

Goal: Tissue repair and scab formation

- New tissue and blood vessels begin to form.
- A scab may form to protect the wound.

Supportive Care:

a. Reapply **natural healing salves** (calendula, comfrey, or manuka honey).
b. Keep wound moist (not wet) to reduce cracking and scar depth.
c. Change dressings daily or as needed.
d. Monitor for infection signs (see below).

3. **Remodeling Stage (Days 10–30+)**

Goal: Strengthening and scar formation

- Skin contracts and reorganizes collagen fibers.
- Color and texture slowly normalize.

Scar-Reducing Support:

a. Gently **massage** the area with **emu oil**, **rosehip oil**, or **vitamin E** once wound is fully closed.
b. Use **silicone tape** or **gel sheets** daily for 12–24 hours to flatten and fade scars.
c. Apply **mineral sunscreen (SPF 30+)** on healing areas to prevent discoloration.

Watch for Signs of Infection:

- Increased redness or swelling after 48 hours
- Yellow, green, or foul-smelling discharge
- Warmth or streaking around the wound
- Fever or fatigue
- Pain increasing rather than improving

Instructions:

If any of these signs are observed, seek prompt medical evaluation. Infection in a child can progress quickly and may require antibiotics.

1. **Colloidal Silver Gel or Spray**

Rationale:

Colloidal silver has natural antibacterial properties that may help reduce bacterial load and inflammation in minor skin wounds. It also supports skin regeneration and may provide a soothing barrier.

Instructions:

a. Gently cleanse the wound with mild soap and water.
b. Apply a thin layer of colloidal silver gel or spray directly to the clean, dry skin.
c. Allow to air dry before dressing with sterile gauze if needed.
d. Reapply 2–3 times per day.

Precaution:

- For external use only.
- Do not use on deep wounds or for prolonged periods without guidance from a healthcare provider.

2. Gentian Violet for Wounds or Superficial Infections

Rationale:

Gentian violet has antiseptic and antibacterial properties that make it useful for small cuts, abrasions, or minor skin infections. It forms a barrier over the skin and may help inhibit the growth of bacteria such as Staphylococcus aureus.

Instructions:

a. Clean the wound thoroughly with mild soap and warm water; pat dry.
b. Dip a sterile cotton swab into the gentian violet solution.
c. Apply a thin, even layer directly onto the wound or infection site.
d. Allow the area to fully dry before applying gauze, if needed.
e. Reapply once daily for no more than 2–4 days.

Precaution:

- Not for use on deep puncture wounds, animal bites, or serious infections.
- Excessive use may delay healing—apply sparingly.
- May cause rash or irritation in sensitive individuals.
- Avoid use in children with eczema or inflamed skin conditions.

3. Manuka Honey or Medical-Grade Raw Honey

Rationale:

Manuka honey is rich in methylglyoxal, a compound with potent antimicrobial and wound-healing properties. It may help fight bacterial infections and maintain a moist healing environment, especially for minor burns, cuts, or infected insect bites.

Instructions:

a. Clean the wound with sterile water or mild soap and pat dry.
b. Apply a small amount of medical-grade Manuka honey directly to the wound.
c. Cover with sterile gauze to hold the honey in place.
d. Change the dressing 1–2 times per day or as needed.

Precaution:

- Do not use near the mouth in infants under 1 year.
- Use only sterilized, medical-grade honey to reduce the risk of contamination.
- Avoid use on large or deep wounds without medical advice.

Scarring and Preventative Measures

Definition:

A scar forms as the skin heals from injury, replacing normal tissue with fibrous tissue. While scarring is a natural part of healing, its appearance can often be minimized with early and consistent care. Children are especially prone to developing visible scars from wounds, burns, and surgical procedures due to active healing and frequent skin injury.

Types of Scars:

- **Flat Scars:** Most common, fade over time
- **Hypertrophic Scars:** Raised, red, thick scars limited to the wound area
- **Keloid Scars:** Extend beyond the original wound; more common in darker skin types
- **Atrophic Scars:** Indented or pitted (e.g., from chickenpox or acne)

When to Begin Scar Care:

Scar prevention should begin once the **skin is fully closed** and free of scabbing or infection. Early care during the remodeling phase (within the first month) is most effective.

Natural Remedies and Topical Treatments to Reduce Scarring

1. Beef Tallow (Grass-Fed)

Rationale:

Beef tallow is rich in fat-soluble vitamins A, D, E, and K and mimics the composition of human sebum. It deeply nourishes the skin, supports barrier repair, and may reduce scarring over time.

Instructions:

a. Apply a small amount of clean-rendered, grass-fed tallow to closed, healed skin.
b. Massage gently into the scar area once or twice daily.
c. Continue use throughout the skin remodeling phase for best results.

Precaution:

- Choose unscented, clean-rendered tallow.
- Patch test before use on sensitive skin.

2. Coconut Oil (Virgin, Cold-Pressed)

Rationale:

Coconut oil has antimicrobial and anti-inflammatory effects and helps hydrate the skin. Regular use may improve softness and reduce the appearance of scars.

Instructions:

a. Apply a thin layer of coconut oil to the scar once or twice daily.
b. Massage gently for 1–2 minutes to stimulate circulation.
c. Use consistently over time for visible results.

Precaution:

- Avoid use if the child has a known coconut allergy.
- May not be suitable for very oily or acne-prone skin.

3. Gentle Massage Therapy

Rationale:

Massage softens scar tissue, reduces adhesions, and promotes local blood flow. When combined with oils, it may help optimize healing and scar remodeling.

Instructions:

a. Use clean fingertips to gently massage the scar in small circular motions.
b. Continue for 1–2 minutes, 1–2 times daily.
c. Pair with moisturizing oils for added benefit.

Precaution:

- Only use on fully healed skin.
- Avoid pressing too firmly, especially in early stages of healing.

4. Rosehip Oil

Rationale:

Rosehip oil is high in essential fatty acids and vitamin A derivatives that may improve skin texture, reduce pigmentation, and support scar fading.

Instructions:

a. Apply 1–2 drops to the scar once daily, preferably in the evening.
b. Gently massage until fully absorbed.
c. Use consistently for several weeks or more.

Precaution:

- Store in a dark glass bottle to prevent oxidation.
- Not for use on open or unhealed skin.

5. Silicone Tape or Silicone Gel Sheets

Rationale:

Silicone-based scar treatments are clinically proven to reduce redness, thickness, and visibility of scars by hydrating the skin and promoting collagen balance.

Instructions:

a. Begin once the wound has fully closed and scabs are gone.
b. Cut the tape or sheet to fit and apply directly over the scar.
c. Wear for 12–24 hours per day.
d. Replace every 3–5 days or per product directions.
e. Continue use for 8–12 weeks or longer if needed.

Precaution:

- Do not use on open or infected wounds.
- Discontinue if redness, rash, or skin reaction occurs.

6. Sun Protection (SPF 30+ Mineral Sunscreen)

Rationale:

UV exposure can darken newly formed scars and increase long-term visibility. Mineral sunscreen protects healing skin from pigmentation changes.

Instructions:

a. Apply mineral-based sunscreen to scars exposed to sunlight.
b. Use protective clothing and wide-brimmed hats for added coverage.
c. Reapply sunscreen every 2 hours during outdoor activity.

Precaution:

- Do not apply sunscreen over open wounds or unhealed scabs.

7. Vitamin E Oil

Rationale:

Vitamin E is an antioxidant that may promote healing and reduce discoloration in mature scars.

Instructions:

a. Use only on closed, fully healed skin.
b. Apply a small amount of vitamin E oil to the scar and massage gently.
c. Use once daily or every other day, depending on skin tolerance.

Precaution:

May cause irritation or allergic reaction in some children—always patch test first.

Burns

Burns are injuries to the skin caused by heat, electricity, friction, radiation, or chemicals. In children, the most common causes are hot liquids (scalds), sunburn, contact with hot surfaces, or accidental exposure to household appliances. Burns are classified by depth and severity, which guides both care and urgency.

Types of Burns:

- **First-Degree Burn:** Affects the outer layer of skin only (epidermis). Skin is red, dry, and painful (e.g., mild sunburn).
- **Second-Degree Burn:** Affects deeper layers (epidermis and part of the dermis). Skin is red or blistered, wet-looking, and very painful.
- **Third-Degree Burn:** Destroys both skin layers and underlying tissue. Skin may appear white, charred, leathery, or numb**. This is a medical emergency.**

Seek Immediate Medical Attention:

- Any burn larger than the size of the child's hand
- Burns involving the **face, hands, genitals, joints, or feet**
- Second- or third-degree burns
- Signs of **infection**: increasing redness, pus, swelling, or fever
- Burns caused by **chemicals, electricity, grease, or fire**
- Burns in **infants under 1 year** or **immunocompromised children**
- Any worsening burn or no improvement within 24–48 hours

Natural Remedies and Comfort Care for Minor Burns (First-Degree or Very Small Second-Degree)

These remedies may be used to support healing in minor, superficial burns only. Do not use natural treatments in place of medical care for more serious burns.

1. Aloe Vera Gel (Pure and Food-Grade)

Rationale:

Aloe vera soothes inflammation, hydrates the skin, and supports regeneration of damaged tissue, making it effective for mild burns.

Instructions:

a. Apply a thin layer of 100% pure aloe vera gel to the affected area.
b. Use 2–3 times daily as needed for soothing and healing.
c. Allow to air dry or cover loosely with a breathable bandage.

Precaution:

- Do not use products containing alcohol, fragrance, or artificial dyes.

2. Avoid Irritants and Friction

Rationale:

Friction and exposure to chemical irritants can delay healing, cause discomfort, and increase the risk of scarring.

Instructions:

a. Dress the child in loose, breathable cotton clothing.
b. Avoid using soaps, creams, or lotions that are not specifically intended for burn care.
c. Keep the area loosely covered if clothing may rub against the burn.

Precaution:

- Avoid rough fabrics and tight-fitting garments until the area has fully healed.

3. Calendula or Chamomile Compress

Rationale:

Calendula and chamomile have anti-inflammatory and soothing properties that may reduce swelling, pain, and redness associated with minor burns.

Instructions:

a. Steep 1–2 teaspoons of dried calendula or chamomile flowers in 1 cup of hot water.
b. Allow the infusion to cool completely.
c. Soak a clean cloth or gauze in the tea and apply to the burn for 10–15 minutes.
d. Repeat 2–3 times daily.

Precaution:

- Ensure the herbal tea is fully cooled before applying.
- Discontinue use if irritation or rash develops.

4. Cool Water Rinse

Rationale:

Immediately cooling the skin after a burn reduces tissue damage, soothes pain, and can slow the progression of the burn.

Instructions:

a. Rinse the burned area under cool (not cold) running water for 10–15 minutes.
b. Alternatively, apply a clean, cool, damp cloth to the area.
c. Pat dry gently with a sterile gauze or clean towel.

Precaution:

- Never use ice directly on the skin, as it can cause further tissue damage.

5. Emu Oil or Coconut Oil (After Healing Phase Begins)

Rationale:

Once the burn has closed and begun healing, emu oil or coconut oil can provide deep moisture and help minimize itching and scarring.

Instructions:

a. Begin use only when the skin is dry, intact, and no longer open.
b. Apply a small amount of oil and massage gently into the healing area once or twice daily.
c. Continue for several weeks during the remodeling phase.

Precaution:

- Avoid use on open wounds or broken skin.
- Use only pure, unscented oils without additives.

6. Hydration and Immune Support

Rationale:

Burn healing increases the body's need for fluids and immune support. Proper hydration and nutrient intake are essential for tissue repair.

Instructions:

a. Encourage frequent fluid intake, including water, bone broth, or herbal teas (see #11 under "Vomiting").
b. Provide antioxidant-rich foods such as berries, carrots, citrus fruits, and leafy greens.
c. Use age-appropriate multivitamins or elderberry syrup to support immune health, if tolerated.

Precaution:

- Avoid sugary drinks and artificial additives.

- Always check supplement safety and dosage by age.

7. Raw Honey (Age 1+)

Rationale:

Raw honey, particularly Manuka honey, is naturally antibacterial and anti-inflammatory. It may accelerate healing and reduce infection risk when applied to minor burns.

Instructions:

a. After cleansing, apply a thin layer of raw honey to the burn.
b. Cover with sterile gauze if needed to protect from clothing or contaminants.
c. Reapply twice daily as needed.

Precaution:

- Do not use in children under 1 year due to the risk of botulism.
- Do not apply to oozing or visibly infected skin.

8. Colloidal Silver

Rationale:

Colloidal silver offers natural antimicrobial protection for superficial burns. It may reduce irritation, prevent bacterial growth, and support the skin's healing process when used in the early stages.

Instructions:

a. First, rinse the burn under cool running water for 10–15 minutes.
b. Pat the area dry gently with a clean cloth or sterile gauze.
c. Spray Sovereign Silver directly onto the burn or apply using a sterile cotton pad.

d. Allow to air dry, or cover with a non-stick bandage if needed.
e. Reapply 2–3 times per day during early healing.

Precaution:

- For external use only.
- Do not use on deep, blistering, or third-degree burns.
- Do not combine with petroleum-based creams during use.
- Always patch test on sensitive skin.
- Discontinue if rash, irritation, or increased redness occurs.

Sunburn

Definition:

Sunburn is a type of first-degree burn caused by overexposure to ultraviolet (UV) rays, typically from sunlight. In children, sunburn can occur quickly—especially with fair skin, during midday sun, or at high altitudes or near water. Repeated sunburns in childhood significantly increase the risk of skin damage and skin cancer later in life.

Causes:

- Prolonged sun exposure without adequate skin protection
- Reflected UV rays from sand, water, snow, or pavement
- Use of photosensitizing medications or essential oils (e.g., citrus oils)
- Thin or wet clothing that allows UV rays to penetrate

Signs and Symptoms:

- Red, warm, painful skin (may take several hours to appear)
- Swelling or tightness of the skin
- Irritability or fussiness in infants or toddlers
- Peeling skin 3–7 days later as healing begins
- In more severe cases: blistering, fever, headache, nausea

Seek Immediate Medical Attention:

- Blistering over a large area of the body
- Signs of dehydration (dry lips, no tears, lethargy)
- Sunburn in a baby under 1 year of age
- Accompanied by fever, vomiting, or confusion
- Swelling of the face or difficulty opening eyes
- Pain that prevents sleeping or worsens after 24 hours

Natural Remedies and Comfort Care for Sunburn (First-Degree)

1. Aloe Vera Gel (100% Pure, Food-Grade)

Rationale:

Aloe vera is a natural anti-inflammatory and hydrator that soothes sun-damaged skin, relieves heat, and supports tissue repair.

Instructions:

a. Apply a thin layer of pure aloe vera gel to clean, dry skin.
b. Use 2–3 times daily or as needed for comfort.
c. Allow the gel to air dry before dressing or applying clothing.

Precaution:

Avoid aloe products that contain alcohol, artificial dyes, or fragrance.

2. Apple Cider Vinegar (ACV) Diluted Spray or Soak

Rationale:

Diluted apple cider vinegar may help restore pH balance and soothe inflamed sunburned skin. It also has mild astringent and cooling effects.

Instructions:

a. Dilute 1 part ACV to 3 parts cool water.
b. Either:

- Spray directly onto sunburned skin using a clean spray bottle, **or**
- Soak a clean cloth in the solution and apply as a compress.

c. Use 1–2 times daily until redness decreases.

Precaution:

- Do not apply to broken, blistered, or highly sensitive skin.
- Discontinue use if stinging or irritation occurs.

3. Chamomile Tea Compress

Rationale:

Chamomile is naturally anti-inflammatory and calming to irritated skin, making it helpful for sunburn relief.

Instructions:

a. Brew a strong cup of chamomile tea and allow it to cool completely.
b. Soak a soft, clean cloth in the tea and wring out.
c. Apply to the sunburned area for 10–15 minutes.
d. Repeat 2–3 times daily as needed.

Precaution:

- Ensure tea is completely cooled before applying.
- Discontinue if rash or reaction develops.

4. Coconut Oil or Emu Oil (Once Redness Calms)

Rationale:

These oils provide deep moisturization, reduce tightness, and help prevent cracking and peeling in the healing stage.

Instructions:

a. Begin use only after initial heat and redness have subsided (typically 24 hours post-burn).
b. Apply a small amount to dry or peeling areas once or twice daily.
c. Massage gently into the skin.

Precaution:

- Do not apply to freshly sunburned or blistered skin.
- Use only pure, unscented oils.

5. Cool Compresses

Rationale:

Cooling the skin helps reduce inflammation, pain, and heat trapped in sunburned tissue.

Instructions:

a. Soak a clean washcloth in cool water.
b. Wring out and apply to the affected area for 10–15 minutes.
c. Repeat every 2–3 hours during the first 24 hours.
d. For added relief, you may add a drop of diluted lavender or chamomile essential oil to the cloth.

Precaution:

- Do not use ice directly on the skin, as it can worsen tissue damage.

6. Hydration and Cooling Foods

Rationale:

Sunburn draws fluids to the skin's surface, increasing risk of dehydration. Internal hydration and nutrient support help the body heal.

Instructions:

a. Offer breast milk, water, bone broth, or homemade electrolyte drinks (see #9 under "Nausea").
b. Include cooling foods such as cucumbers, melons, oranges, and leafy greens.

c. Avoid processed, fried, or salty foods that can worsen dehydration.

Precaution:

- Monitor for signs of dehydration, especially in younger children.

7. Lukewarm Baths with Baking Soda or Oatmeal

Rationale:

These ingredients soothe itching and inflammation while softening dry, sun-damaged skin.

Instructions:

a. Fill a bathtub with lukewarm water (not hot).
b. Add ¼ cup baking soda **or** ½ cup colloidal oatmeal.
c. Let the child soak for 10–15 minutes.
d. Gently pat skin dry—do not rub.

Precaution:

- Always test water temperature before placing child in the bath.

8. Loose Cotton Clothing and Rest

Rationale:

Soft, breathable clothing protects damaged skin from further irritation and supports the body's healing process.

Instructions:

a. Dress the child in loose, light-colored cotton clothing.
b. Keep the child indoors or in shaded areas until the skin fully recovers.
c. Encourage rest and low-activity play during recovery.

Precaution:

- Avoid synthetic or tight clothing until the skin has healed.

Sunburn Prevention Tips

- Apply **mineral sunscreen (SPF 30+)** 15–30 minutes before sun exposure and reapply every 2 hours.
- Avoid sun exposure between **10 a.m. and 4 p.m.**, especially in summer.
- Use **wide-brimmed hats**, **UV-protective clothing**, and **sunglasses** outdoors.
- Remember: **Cloud cover and water do not prevent UV exposure**—sun protection is still necessary.

Bug Bites, Insect Stings, and Jellyfish Stings

This section includes common skin reactions from mosquitoes, ants, bees, wasps, spiders, and jellyfish. Reactions vary from mild itching and swelling to more serious allergic responses. Prompt and supportive care can greatly reduce discomfort, prevent complications, and promote healing.

General Signs and Symptoms:

- Local redness, swelling, and tenderness
- Itching or burning sensation
- Raised bump, welt, or small puncture
- In jellyfish stings: whip-like welts, severe burning or stinging

Seek Immediate Medical Attention:

- Difficulty breathing, facial or throat swelling, hives, or wheezing
- Sting inside the mouth or near the eyes
- Rapid spreading redness, signs of infection, or fever
- Jellyfish sting with severe pain, vomiting, difficulty breathing
- Sting from a black widow, brown recluse, or unknown spider
- Any bite or sting in a child under 1 year

Natural Remedies for Bug Bites

1. Aloe Vera Gel

Rationale:

Aloe vera is cooling, hydrating, and anti-inflammatory. It helps soothe itching and reduces redness.

Instructions:

a. Apply a small amount of pure aloe vera gel directly to the bite.

b. Reapply 2–3 times daily as needed.

2. Apple Cider Vinegar Dab

Rationale:

Apple cider vinegar helps balance the skin's pH and reduce itching and inflammation.

Instructions:

a. Dilute apple cider vinegar 1:1 with water.
b. Dab the solution onto the bite using a clean cotton ball.
c. Reapply as needed throughout the day.

Precaution:

Do not apply to broken skin or open wounds.

3. Arnica Gel or Cream

Rationale:

Arnica reduces swelling, bruising, and tenderness around the bite area.

Instructions:

a. Apply a small amount of arnica gel to the affected area.
b. Use 2–3 times daily until swelling and discomfort resolve.

Precaution:

- Do not apply to open or broken skin.

4. Baking Soda Paste

Rationale:

Baking soda neutralizes toxins and calms itch and irritation.

Instructions:

a. Mix 1 tablespoon of baking soda with a few drops of water to form a paste.
b. Apply to the bite and leave on for 10–15 minutes.
c. Rinse off and reapply 2–3 times daily as needed.

5. Calendula or Chamomile Cream

Rationale:

Both herbs have anti-inflammatory and skin-soothing properties that help relieve itching and irritation.

Instructions:

a. Apply a thin layer of calendula or chamomile cream to the bite.
b. Use 2–3 times per day.

6. Cold Compress

Rationale:

Cold application reduces inflammation, pain, and itching by constricting blood vessels.

Instructions:

a. Apply a cool, damp washcloth or wrapped ice pack to the bite for 5–10 minutes.
b. Repeat every few hours as needed.

Precaution:

- Do not place ice directly on the skin.

7. Essential Oils (Age 2+)

Rationale:

Lavender and tea tree oils have anti-inflammatory and antimicrobial properties that reduce itch and prevent infection.

Instructions:

a. Dilute 1 drop of essential oil in 1 teaspoon of carrier oil (e.g., coconut or olive).
b. Apply directly to the bite up to 3 times daily.

Precaution:

- Not for use in children under age 2.
- Avoid contact with eyes and mucous membranes.

8. Honey (Age 1+)

Rationale:

Raw honey has antibacterial and anti-inflammatory effects that help soothe and heal irritated bites.

Instructions:

a. Dab a small amount of raw honey on the bite.
b. Let air dry or cover loosely with gauze.
c. Reapply 2–3 times daily.

Precaution:

Do not use in children under 1 year due to botulism risk.

Insect Stings (Bees, Wasps, Hornets, Fire Ants)

Definition:

Stings from insects such as bees and wasps can cause immediate pain, swelling, and allergic reactions. Prompt treatment helps reduce discomfort and prevent complications.

Seek Immediate Medical Attention

- If a child experiences any of the following:
- Difficulty breathing or swallowing
- Swelling of the lips, tongue, or face
- Dizziness or fainting
- Widespread hives or rash
- Vomiting or rapid heart rate

Call 911 or go to the nearest emergency room.

First Step for Bee Stings

Remove the Stinger

Instructions:

a. Use a flat-edged object (like a credit card) to gently scrape off the stinger.
b. Avoid using tweezers or fingers to squeeze the stinger.

Natural Remedies for Insect Stings

1. Arnica (Topical or Homeopathic)

Rationale:

Reduces pain, inflammation, and bruising at the sting site.

Instructions:

a. Apply arnica gel to the cleaned sting site 2–3 times daily.
b. For added support, give arnica 30C pellets (2–3 pellets under tongue every 4–6 hours).

2. Baking Soda Paste (for Bee Stings)

Rationale:

Bee venom is acidic; baking soda helps neutralize it and soothe the area.

Instructions:

a. Mix baking soda with water to form a paste.
b. Apply to the sting for 10–15 minutes, then rinse.
c. Repeat as needed.

3. Cold Compress

Rationale:

Provides quick pain relief and minimizes swelling.

Instructions:

a. Apply a cool cloth or wrapped ice pack to the sting site for 10–15 minutes.
b. Repeat every few hours as needed.

4. Lavender Essential Oil (Age 2+)

Rationale:

Lavender oil soothes burning and helps reduce inflammation.

Instructions:

a. Dilute 1 drop of lavender oil in 1 teaspoon of carrier oil.
b. Apply gently to the sting area.

Precaution:

- Do not apply undiluted oil to children's skin.

5. Meat Tenderizer Paste

Rationale:

Contains the enzyme papain, which may help break down sting venom proteins.

Instructions:

a. Mix meat tenderizer powder with water to make a paste.
b. Apply to the sting for 10–15 minutes, then rinse.
c. Repeat once or twice as needed.

6. Onion Slice Compress

Rationale:

Onion has natural antihistamine and anti-inflammatory properties that help reduce swelling and pain.

Instructions:

a. Place a fresh onion slice directly over the sting.
b. Leave on for 10–15 minutes.
c. Discard after use.

7. Vinegar Dab (for Wasp Stings)

Rationale:

Wasp venom is alkaline; vinegar helps neutralize it and relieve burning.

Instructions:

a. Dilute vinegar with equal parts water.
b. Dab gently onto the sting site using a cotton ball.
c. Repeat every few hours as needed.

Jellyfish Stings

Definition:

Jellyfish stings can cause burning pain, redness, welts, and in some cases, systemic reactions. Prompt neutralization and gentle removal of tentacles is essential.

Seek Immediate Medical Attention

If the child experiences:

- Trouble breathing or chest pain
- Dizziness or fainting
- Severe or spreading rash
- Nausea, vomiting, or muscle cramping
- Stings covering a large area or near the eyes

Immediate First Aid for Jellyfish Stings

1. Rinse with Vinegar

Rationale:

Neutralizes stinging cells (nematocysts) and prevents further toxin release.

Instructions:

a. Pour white vinegar directly over the affected area for 30–60 seconds.
b. If vinegar is unavailable, rinse with seawater—never fresh water.

2. Remove Tentacles

Instructions:

a. Using tweezers or gloved hands, carefully remove any visible tentacles.
b. Rinse again with vinegar afterward.

Soothing Remedies for Jellyfish Stings

3. Arnica (Topical or Oral)

(See Remedy #1 under "Insect Stings")

4. Baking Soda Paste

(See Remedy #2 under "Insect Stings")

5. Meat Tenderizer Paste

(See Remedy #5 under "Insect Stings")

- Use for up to 20 minutes.

6. Warm Water Soak

Rationale:

Heat deactivates venom proteins and relieves muscle pain.

Instructions:

a. Soak the affected area in warm (not hot) water for 20–30 minutes.
b. If immersion is not possible, use warm compresses.

CHAPTER 09

FEVER

This section is for educational purposes only. The remedies listed are intended to support comfort and wellness and should not be used as a substitute for professional medical advice. Always consult your child's healthcare provider for diagnosis and treatment.

Fever

Fever is defined as a temporary elevation in body temperature, often due to the body's natural response to infection or inflammation. In children, a rectal temperature of **100.4°F (38°C)** or higher is considered a fever. Though it can be alarming to parents, fever itself is a sign that the immune system is working and is not inherently harmful.

Causes:

- Viral infections (e.g., cold, flu, RSV, roseola)
- Bacterial infections (e.g., strep throat, UTI, ear infection)
- Teething (mild fevers only)
- Recent vaccinations
- Overheating (not the same as true infection-related fever)

Signs and Symptoms:

- Warm or flushed skin
- Sweating or chills
- Fatigue, fussiness, or crying
- Decreased appetite
- Rapid breathing or heart rate
- Body aches or sensitivity to light
- Irritability or sleep changes

Seek Immediate Medical Attention:

- Fever in an infant under 3 months of age (≥100.4°F / 38°C)
- Fever over 104°F (40°C) in any child
- Seizure activity or stiff neck
- Difficulty breathing or unresponsiveness
- Persistent vomiting or refusal to drink
- Fever lasting more than 3 days
- Rash with purple or bruise-like spots
- Lethargy, poor eye contact, or inconsolable crying

Understanding the Benefits of Fever

Fever is the body's natural response to infection. It is not an illness itself, but a powerful immune mechanism designed to fight off bacteria and viruses. A rise in temperature helps:

- Slow the growth of invading pathogens
- Activate white blood cells and immune defenses
- Signal the body to rest and heal

While it may feel alarming, most fevers are not dangerous, especially in otherwise healthy children. Many pediatric fevers resolve on their own within 2–3 days with rest, hydration, and comfort care.

When to Be Concerned
You should seek immediate medical attention if your child has:

- A fever in an infant under 3 months (≥100.4°F / 38°C)
- A fever over 104°F (40°C) in any age group
- Persistent fever lasting more than 72 hours
- Difficulty breathing, severe lethargy, or unresponsiveness
- A seizure or a fever accompanied by a stiff neck, severe headache, or rash
- Refusal to drink, signs of dehydration, or persistent vomiting

Always trust your instincts—if your child seems unusually ill, do not hesitate to contact your pediatrician or go to the ER.

Accuracy of Thermometers

Accurate temperature measurement is an essential part of assessing a child's health. Fever is often the first sign of infection or inflammation, and using the correct type of thermometer in the appropriate location is critical for reliable readings.

Most Accurate Method:
Rectal thermometers provide the most accurate reading of

a child's core body temperature. This is especially important in infants and young children where fever can be a critical indicator of illness.

Common Types of Thermometers:

- Rectal Thermometers: Most accurate; recommended for infants under 3 years old.
- Oral Thermometers: Accurate for older children who can hold the thermometer under the tongue without movement.
- Axillary (Armpit) Thermometers: Less accurate but may be used for quick screening.
- Tympanic (Ear) Thermometers: Convenient, but may give inaccurate readings if not placed correctly or if earwax is present.
- Temporal Artery (Forehead) Thermometers: Non-invasive and quick, but can be less reliable depending on the device and placement.

Important Note:
Read all manufacturer instructions carefully before using any thermometer. Do not use the same thermometer for rectal and oral readings. Label them clearly to avoid cross-contamination.

How to Take a Rectal Temperature Safely

Rationale:

Rectal temperature gives the most direct measure of internal body heat and is considered the gold standard in infants. It is especially useful in evaluating newborns or when fever must be confirmed with certainty.

Instructions:

a. Wash your hands and clean the thermometer tip with rubbing alcohol or warm,, soapy water.

b. Label the thermometer as "rectal only" to prevent confusion.
c. Apply a small amount of water-based lubricant (e.g., petroleum jelly) to the tip of the thermometer.
d. Lay the baby on their back with legs lifted gently or position them face-down across your lap.
e. Gently insert the thermometer into the rectum no more than 1/2 to 1 inch (about 1.25 to 2.5 cm) depending on the child's size.
f. Hold the thermometer steady and keep your hand on the child's bottom to prevent movement.
g. Wait for the thermometer to beep or finish reading (typically 10–30 seconds).
h. Carefully remove the thermometer, clean it thoroughly, and record the temperature.

Precaution:

- Do not insert the thermometer deeply. Insertion deeper than 1 inch increases the risk of rectal perforation.
- Always use a thermometer with a flexible tip and wide base to prevent over-insertion.
- Never force the thermometer into the rectum. If resistance is felt, stop immediately.
- Disinfect after each use and store separately from oral thermometers.
- Seek immediate medical care if you suspect injury or bleeding after taking a rectal temperature.

Natural Remedies and Comfort Care for Fever

1. **Cold Sock Method (Warming Sock Treatment)**

Rationale:

This hydrotherapy method supports immune response and restful sleep by drawing circulation away from the head and promoting systemic regulation.

Instructions:

a. Soak a pair of thin cotton socks in cold water and wring out completely.
b. Put the cold, wet socks on the child's feet.
c. Immediately cover with a second pair of dry wool or thick cotton socks.
d. Bundle the child warmly in bed and leave socks on overnight or until fully dry.

Precaution:

- Only use in children who are warm overall.
- Do not use in infants under 6 months or if the child is chilled or shivering.

2. **Cool Compress to Neck, Armpits, and Groin**

Rationale:

Applying cool (not cold) compresses to areas with major blood vessels helps reduce core temperature safely and naturally.

Instructions:

a. Soak soft cloths in cool water and wring out gently.
b. Apply to the back of the neck, armpits, and groin area.
c. Rotate every 10–15 minutes as needed.
d. Continue until the fever begins to drop or the child feels more comfortable.

Precaution:

- Do not use ice or very cold water.
- Stop immediately if the child becomes chilled.

3. Herbal Teas for Immune and Fever Support (Age 2+)

Rationale:

Mild herbal teas such as elderflower, chamomile, and yarrow promote sweating and support the immune response during fevers.

Instructions:

a. Steep 1 teaspoon of dried herb in 1 cup of hot water for 10 minutes.
b. Cool completely before offering.
c. Offer 1–2 tablespoons at a time, 2–3 times per day.

Precaution:

- Do not give herbal teas to infants under 2 years.
- Avoid licorice and strong herbal blends in children under 6.

4. Hydration with Electrolyte Support

Rationale:

Fever leads to increased fluid loss. Maintaining hydration helps regulate temperature and prevents dehydration-related complications.

Instructions:

a. Offer breast milk, bone broth, diluted fruit juice, or a homemade electrolyte drink (see Remedy #9 under "Nausea").
b. Encourage small, frequent sips throughout the day.
c. Use a dropper, syringe, or spoon for infants if needed.

Precaution:

- Avoid sugary drinks and sodas.
- Monitor for signs of dehydration (dry lips, no tears, sunken eyes, reduced urination).

5. Lukewarm Epsom Salt Bath with Essential Oils

Rationale:

A lukewarm bath gently lowers body temperature while Epsom salt supports detoxification and muscle relaxation. Lavender or chamomile oil offers added soothing benefits.

Instructions:

a. Fill the tub with lukewarm water (never cold or hot).
b. Add ½ cup Epsom salt for toddlers or 1 cup for older children.
c. Mix in 1–2 drops of lavender or chamomile essential oil, pre-diluted in 1 tablespoon of carrier oil.
d. Let the child soak for 10–15 minutes under supervision.
e. Dry gently and dress in breathable, loose-fitting cotton clothing.

Precaution:

- Never use hot water during a fever.
- Do not use peppermint oil in children under 6.
- Always supervise young children in the bath.

6. Peppermint Essential Oil Compress (Age 6+ Only)

Rationale:

Peppermint provides natural cooling relief and may ease headache or discomfort associated with fever.

Instructions:

a. Add 1 drop of peppermint oil to a bowl of cool water.
b. Soak a clean washcloth in the mixture and wring out.
c. Apply to the forehead or back of the neck.
d. Reapply as needed.

Precaution:

- Avoid use on the face of children under age 6.

- Never apply undiluted essential oils directly to skin.

7. Rest and Light Clothing

Rationale:

Allowing the body to rest conserves energy for healing. Light clothing helps regulate temperature without trapping heat.

Instructions:

a. Keep the child in a quiet, cool environment with minimal stimulation.
b. Dress in breathable cotton pajamas or clothing.
c. Avoid heavy blankets or bundling.

Precaution:

- Do not underdress or expose the child to cold air.
- Adjust clothing based on comfort and room temperature.

8. Vinegar Socks for Fever

Rationale:

Vinegar socks are a traditional remedy used to gently draw heat from the body through the feet, supporting temperature regulation via evaporative cooling and improved circulation.

Instructions:

a. Mix equal parts apple cider vinegar and cool water (e.g., ½ cup each) in a small bowl.
b. Soak a pair of thin cotton socks in the solution and wring out until damp.
c. Place the damp vinegar socks on the child's feet.
d. Cover with a second pair of dry wool or thick cotton socks.
e. Let the child rest for 30–60 minutes.

f. Reapply every few hours if fever persists, checking that the child remains warm and comfortable.

Precaution:

- Do not use if the child has cold feet, chills, or is shivering.
- Discontinue if any skin irritation or rash develops.
- Monitor closely to ensure comfort and warmth.

Febrile Seizures

Febrile seizures are convulsions that can occur in children due to a sudden rise in body temperature, most often between the ages of 6 months and 5 years. They can be frightening but are typically brief and harmless.

Signs of a Febrile Seizure:

- Sudden loss of consciousness
- Muscle stiffening followed by rhythmic jerking
- Eyes rolling back
- Drooling or foaming at the mouth
- Lasts less than 5 minutes (in most cases)
- May be followed by drowsiness or confusion

What to Do at Home During a Febrile Seizure:

a. Remain calm and keep the child safe.
b. Gently lay the child on their side on a soft, flat surface away from sharp objects.
c. Do **not** restrain movements or place anything in the child's mouth.
d. Note the **duration** of the seizure.
e. Loosen tight clothing and do not attempt to bring the fever down during the seizure.
f. After the seizure stops, monitor breathing and responsiveness.

Call 911 or go to the nearest ER if:

- The seizure lasts longer than **5 minutes**
- The child has **trouble breathing** or turns blue
- Your child is **under 6 months old**
- The seizure occurs **without a fever**
- Your child does not regain full consciousness after the event
- It is the **first seizure** or you are unsure what is happening

Follow-Up:

Most children with a febrile seizure do not develop epilepsy or other long-term issues. Still, any seizure should be followed by a visit to a healthcare provider to rule out underlying causes and receive personalized guidance.

CHAPTER 10

IMMUNE SUPPORT

This section is for educational purposes only. The remedies listed are intended to support comfort and wellness and should not be used as a substitute for professional medical advice. Always consult your child's healthcare provider for diagnosis and treatment.

Immune Support

This chapter provides practical, natural tools to support and strengthen your child's developing immune system. These approaches are not meant to replace medical care but to work alongside it—enhancing recovery, reducing the severity of illness, and building long-term immune resilience through nutrition, daily habits, and holistic care.

The Purpose of Immune Support in Childhood

Children's immune systems are constantly developing, learning to respond to viruses, bacteria, and environmental stressors. Gentle nourishment—rather than suppressing every symptom—helps build lifelong resilience. Illness is a natural part of immune learning, and with the right tools, parents can support their child's recovery while minimizing unnecessary discomfort.

1. Additional Immune-Boosting Lifestyle Habits

Rationale:

Everyday habits play a critical role in strengthening a child's immune system and building resilience to illness.

Instructions:

a. Prioritize consistent sleep and bedtime routines (see Sleep Chapter for details).
b. Encourage outdoor movement, yoga, or dancing to promote circulation.
c. Reduce intake of sugar and processed foods to preserve immune cell function.
d. Support gut health with fermented foods or probiotics, especially after antibiotics.
e. Provide emotional comfort with nurturing routines, creative play, and quality time.

f. Maintain steady hydration using water, herbal teas, or broth throughout the day.

Precaution:

- Adjust strategies based on your child's developmental stage and temperament.

2. "Amish Amoxicillin" Immune Tonic

Rationale:

This raw, blended tonic includes garlic, ginger, pineapple, turmeric, lemon, and honey—known for their antiviral, antibacterial, and anti-inflammatory effects.

Instructions:

a. Blend juice of 1 lemon, 1 onion, 1 thumb of ginger, 3–4 garlic cloves, 1 tbsp turmeric, 1 tsp black pepper, 1 tbsp cayenne, 3 tbsp Manuka honey, 1 whole pineapple, and ¼ cup apple cider vinegar.
b. Store in a sealed glass jar in the refrigerator.

Dosage:

Children over 1: ½–1 tsp up to 3x daily.

Adults: 1 tbsp 2–3x daily.

Precaution:

- Avoid in children sensitive to garlic, pineapple, or strong spice.
- Start with small doses to assess tolerance.

3. Choosing High-Quality Supplements

Rationale:

High-quality supplements improve absorption and reduce exposure to additives or ineffective forms of nutrients.

Instructions:

a. Choose third-party tested brands that verify purity and potency.
b. Use liposomal forms of vitamin C, glutathione, and curcumin for better absorption.
c. Opt for liquid, powder, or chewable forms for children.
d. Avoid artificial dyes, flavors, or fillers.
e. Refrigerate probiotics unless labeled as shelf-stable.

Precaution:

Consult a healthcare provider before giving supplements to children under 2 or for long-term use.

4. Elderberry and Spice Immune Syrup

Rationale:

Elderberries are rich in antioxidants and antiviral compounds. Combined with warming spices and raw honey, this syrup supports the immune system and soothes the throat.

Instructions:

a. Simmer ½ cup dried elderberries, 2 cups water, 1 tsp cinnamon, 1 tsp ginger, and 3–4 cloves for 30–45 minutes.
b. Strain and cool slightly.
c. Stir in ½ cup raw honey.
d. Store in a sealed glass bottle in the refrigerator.

Dosage:

Children over 1: ½ tsp daily for prevention or every 3 hours when ill.

Adults: 1 tbsp daily or every 3 hours when ill.

Precaution:

- Do not give honey to children under 12 months.
- Discontinue if rash or digestive upset occurs.

5. Fire Cider Immunity Tonic (Age 5+)

Rationale:

This vinegar-based remedy uses garlic, horseradish, cayenne, and lemon to support circulation, break up mucus, and activate immune defenses.

Instructions:

a. Combine ½ cup apple cider vinegar, 1 chopped onion, 3 garlic cloves, 1 hot pepper or ½ tsp cayenne, 1 tbsp horseradish, 1 tsp turmeric, and juice of 1 lemon in a jar.
b. Cover and infuse at room temperature for 24 hours.
c. Strain and stir in ½ cup raw honey.
d. Store in the refrigerator and shake before use.

Dosage:

Children over 5: ½ tsp diluted in water daily or during illness.

Teens/Adults: 1 tbsp daily or every 4 hours during symptoms.

Precaution:

- Not for children under 5.
- Avoid in children with spice sensitivities or reflux.

6. Grounding for Immune and Nervous System Regulation

Rationale:

Direct contact with the Earth's surface may help reduce inflammation, balance cortisol levels, and enhance immune function.

Instructions:

a. Let children walk barefoot on grass, soil, sand, or stone for 15–30 minutes daily.
b. Lie on a blanket outdoors or touch trees, rocks, or soil with bare hands.
c. Use grounding mats indoors if outdoor access is limited.
d. Combine grounding with quiet activities such as nature journaling or stretching.

Precaution:

- Supervise young children and avoid sharp, hot, or unsafe surfaces.

7. Homemade Vitamin C Paste or Syrup (Citrus-Infused)

Rationale:

This citrus remedy provides whole-food vitamin C and bioflavonoids. Baking or steaming citrus fruits enhances absorption while reducing acidity.

Instructions for Paste:

a. Wash and quarter 2–3 organic citrus fruits (e.g., oranges, lemons, grapefruit).
b. Bake or steam at 250°F for 30–45 minutes.
c. Blend the entire fruit (peel included) into a smooth paste.
d. Strain if desired, or leave unstrained for texture.
e. Store in a glass jar in the fridge for up to 5 days.

Serving Suggestion:

Add 1–2 tsp to warm water, herbal tea, or smoothies for children over 1.

Instructions for Syrup:

a. Follow steps a–c above, then strain the blended mixture.
b. Warm gently (do not boil), then stir in ½ cup raw honey.
c. Cool completely and store in a sterilized bottle for up to 2 weeks.

Serving Suggestion:

Give 1–2 tsp daily during cold/flu season or every few hours during illness.

Precaution:

- Do not give honey to infants under 12 months.
- Use only organic citrus.
- Introduce slowly in children with reflux or citrus sensitivity.

8. Immune-Boosting Superfoods for Children

Rationale:

Superfoods provide concentrated nutrients that support immunity, tissue repair, and natural detoxification.

Recommended Superfoods:

Sea Moss: Natural multivitamin with 90+ trace minerals. Blend into smoothies or applesauce.

Colostrum: Contains antibodies and growth factors. Use in pediatric supplement form.

Tart Cherry Juice: High in antioxidants and melatonin—promotes healing and sleep.

Bone Broth: Rich in collagen, glutamine, and electrolytes for gut and immune health.

Elderberries: Potent antiviral; use in syrups or lozenges.

Moringa Powder: Vitamin-rich; add to smoothies or foods.

Garlic: Antiviral and antibacterial; best raw or lightly cooked.

Goji Berries: Nutrient-dense; soak and add to cereal or smoothies.

Raw Honey (Age 1+): Soothes throat and has antimicrobial effects.

Bee Propolis: Supports respiratory immunity; use as spray or drops.

Turmeric (with black pepper): Anti-inflammatory and detoxifying.

Precaution:

- Introduce new foods gradually.
- Use age-appropriate amounts.
- Avoid honey in children under 1.
- Monitor for allergies or food sensitivities.

9. Colloidal Silver Nasal Spray

Rationale:

Colloidal silver helps reduce nasal microbial load and may prevent viral replication at the point of entry.

Instructions:

- Shake gently before use.
- Tilt the child's head back and spray 1–2 times per nostril, up to 3 times daily.

Precaution:

- For ages 1+.
- Do not use longer than 10 days.
- Do not share spray nozzles between users.
- Avoid in children with known silver sensitivity.

10. Sunlight for Immune Activation

Rationale:

Sunlight is the body's natural source of vitamin D and supports immune regulation, serotonin balance, and circadian rhythm.

Instructions:

a. Encourage 15–30 minutes of sun exposure on the face, arms, or legs daily.
b. Favor morning or late afternoon sun.
c. Allow brief exposure before applying sunscreen.

Precaution:

- Avoid sunburn—use hats and natural sunblock for longer exposure.
- Keep babies shaded and hydrated in warm weather.

11. Zinc Nasal Swabs (Age 5+)

Rationale:

Topical zinc applied to nasal passages may help block early-stage viral replication.

Instructions:

a. Use only child-specific zinc nasal swabs.
b. Gently apply to the inner nostril lining twice daily during early illness.

Precaution:

- Do not insert deeply.
- Avoid use beyond 3 days.
- Discontinue if burning or irritation occurs.

Essential Oils for Children

Common Uses and Safe Selection

Essential oils are highly concentrated plant extracts that can provide therapeutic benefits when used carefully and in appropriate dilution. Many essential oils have calming, antimicrobial, or decongestant properties that support comfort and wellness in children. When used properly, they can be incorporated into diffusers, massage oils, baths, or topical blends.

Common Essential Oils and Their Qualities

1. **Lavender (Lavandula angustifolia)**

- Calming, anti-inflammatory, promotes restful sleep
- Can soothe skin irritation and reduce minor pain
- Safe for most ages when diluted

2. **Roman Chamomile (Chamaemelum nobile)**

- Gentle and calming for restlessness, teething, and colic
- Supports skin healing and reduces inflammation

3. **Tea Tree (Melaleuca alternifolia)**

- Antifungal, antibacterial, and antiviral
- Useful for minor cuts, skin infections, and insect bites
- Not recommended for use on children under age 2

4. **Eucalyptus (Eucalyptus radiata – NOT globulus for children)**

- Helps relieve nasal congestion and respiratory symptoms
- Age 2+ in diluted form; use in diffuser or chest rub

5. **Frankincense (Boswellia carterii)**

- Anti-inflammatory, grounding, immune-supportive

- Supports respiratory health and emotional regulation

6. **Lemon (Citrus limon)**

- Uplifting and cleansing; supports immune function
- Antibacterial and purifying for room sprays
- Phototoxic – avoid sun exposure on applied areas

7. **Peppermint (Mentha piperita)**

- Cooling and anti-nausea
- Can ease headaches or digestive upset
- Not for children under age 6 or near the face of infants

8. **Sweet Orange (Citrus sinensis)**

- Cheerful and uplifting
- Supports digestion and emotional balance
- Gentle enough for most children in diffuser blends

9. **Cedarwood (Cedrus atlantica)**

- Calming and grounding; supports sleep and focus
- May help with skin issues such as eczema

10. **Geranium (Pelargonium graveolens)**

- Supports hormone balance and skin repair
- Antimicrobial and soothing for rashes or minor wounds

Selecting High-Quality Essential Oils

Rationale:

Pure, high-grade essential oils are critical to avoid adverse reactions, especially in children. Many products on the market are adulterated with synthetic chemicals or diluted with inferior ingredients.

How to Choose a Quality Essential Oil:

a. Look for oils labeled as **100% pure essential oil** with the Latin (botanical) name on the label.
b. Choose oils from reputable companies that offer **GC/MS (Gas Chromatography/Mass Spectrometry) test reports** verifying chemical composition and purity.
c. Select oils packaged in **dark glass bottles** (amber or cobalt blue) with tightly sealed lids to protect from light and air degradation.
d. Avoid products labeled "fragrance oil," "perfume oil," or simply "aromatherapy oil," as these may contain synthetic additives.
e. Check for **country of origin, harvest method, and distillation date**, which high-quality companies will often provide.

Signs of Low-Quality Oils:

- No Latin name or transparency on the label
- Strongly perfumed or synthetic smell
- Sold in plastic or clear bottles
- Suspiciously low pricing for rare oils (e.g., rose, sandalwood)
- No batch number, testing information, or sourcing transparency

Cautions When Using Essential Oils in Children:

- Always **dilute essential oils** in a carrier oil (such as coconut, olive, or jojoba oil) before applying to the skin.
- **Avoid internal use** of essential oils in children unless directed by a licensed healthcare provider trained in essential oil safety.
- **Never apply undiluted oils** to a child's skin.
- **Do not apply near the face or chest** of infants under 1 year, especially eucalyptus or peppermint.
- Use caution with **citrus oils** (like lemon) on the skin before sun exposure due to phototoxicity.

CHAPTER 11

SLEEP

This section is for educational purposes only. The remedies listed are intended to support comfort and wellness and should not be used as a substitute for professional medical advice. Always consult your child's healthcare provider for diagnosis and treatment.

Pediatric Sleep Support

Creating a healthy sleep routine is vital for a child's physical, emotional, and cognitive development. Children thrive on consistency and comfort, and a predictable sleep environment helps regulate circadian rhythms, reduces nighttime anxiety, and supports restful, restorative sleep.

This section offers practical guidance for establishing a safe and calming bedtime environment, along with evidence-informed natural strategies that may promote sleep in children. Remedies should always be age-appropriate and used with care.

Creating a Soothing and Safe Sleep Environment

A calming sleep space helps ease the transition from wakefulness to rest. Children, especially infants and toddlers, need a secure, predictable setting to feel relaxed and fall asleep more easily.

1. Blankets for Older Children (Age 2+)

Rationale:

Soft, breathable blankets can offer warmth and a sense of comfort, often becoming part of a child's emotional sleep association as they grow.

Instructions:

a. Select lightweight materials such as cotton, muslin, or bamboo.
b. Allow the child to choose a preferred blanket to foster attachment.
c. Use breathable fabrics that do not trap excess heat.
d. For toddlers who move during sleep, tuck the blanket under the mattress to minimize tangling.

Precaution:

- Do not use loose blankets in children under age 2 due to suffocation risk.
- Wash regularly to maintain hygiene and reduce allergens.

2. Chamomile Tea (Age 1+)

Rationale:

Chamomile is a gentle herbal remedy known for calming the nervous system, easing mild anxiety, and promoting sleep.

Instructions:

a. Steep 1 teaspoon of dried chamomile flowers in 1 cup of hot water for 5–10 minutes.
b. Cool completely before offering.
c. Give 1–2 tablespoons to toddlers or up to ½ cup for older children before bedtime.

Precaution:

- Not suitable for infants under 12 months.
- Avoid use in children with ragweed allergies.

3. Comfort Objects

Rationale:

Soft items like stuffed animals or blankets help provide emotional security and smooth transitions into sleep.

Instructions:

a. Choose age-appropriate, safe comfort items.
b. For infants under 12 months, avoid loose objects in the crib.
c. Ensure items are free of strings or small parts.

4. Essential Oil Diffuser (Age 2+)

Rationale:

Aromatherapy with calming essential oils such as lavender or chamomile may ease bedtime resistance and promote relaxation.

Instructions:

a. Add 2–4 drops of essential oil to a cool-mist diffuser filled with water.
b. Run the diffuser for 30–60 minutes before bedtime.

Precaution:

- Only use child-safe, high-quality essential oils.
- Avoid peppermint and eucalyptus in young children.
- Ensure proper ventilation.

5. Gentle Pressure Point Therapy (Age 3+)

Rationale:

Light acupressure and massage can help calm the body, reduce restlessness, and activate the parasympathetic nervous system.

Instructions:

a. Gently massage areas such as the soles of the feet, between the eyebrows, or inner wrists.
b. Use slow, circular motions with a carrier oil like coconut or olive oil.
c. Perform for 3–5 minutes during the bedtime routine.

Precaution:

- Use only light pressure appropriate to the child's size.
- Discontinue if the child appears overstimulated or uncomfortable.

6. Humidifier (Cool Mist)

Rationale:

Moist air helps ease nighttime coughing, soothe dry sinuses, and support restful breathing.

Instructions:

a. Use a cool-mist humidifier during dry weather or illness.
b. Clean thoroughly and change the water daily to prevent mold.

7. Lemon Balm Tea (Age 1+)

Rationale:

Lemon balm (Melissa officinalis) calms the nervous system and may improve sleep quality in children with irritability or restlessness.

Instructions:

a. Steep 1 teaspoon of dried lemon balm in 1 cup of hot water for 5–7 minutes.
b. Cool completely.
c. Offer 1–2 tablespoons to toddlers or up to ½ cup for older children before bed.

Precaution:

- Avoid in children with thyroid disorders unless approved by a provider.
- Do not exceed daily use without medical advice.

8. Lighting and Nightlights

Rationale:

Warm, dim lighting signals the brain that it's time to wind down and enhances natural melatonin production.

Instructions:

a. Use amber-toned or red-spectrum nightlights if a night light is needed.
b. Avoid screens and bright overhead lights 1–2 hours before bedtime.
c. Keep the sleeping area as dark as possible during the night.

9. Magnesium (Age 2+, Pediatric Formulas)

Rationale:

Magnesium supports muscle relaxation and nervous system regulation, promoting restful sleep.

Instructions:

a. Use age-appropriate magnesium supplements or bath soaks.
b. For baths: Add ½ cup magnesium flakes to warm water and soak for 15 minutes before bed.
c. For oral use: Follow pediatric dosing or consult a provider.

Precaution:

- May cause loose stools if overdosed orally.
- Do not give oral magnesium to children under 2 without supervision.

10. Melatonin (Use with Caution, Age 3+)

Rationale:

Melatonin is a sleep-regulating hormone that may benefit children with sleep disorders, autism, or significant bedtime struggles when used short-term.

Instructions:

a. Use pediatric doses only (typically 0.5–1 mg).
b. Administer 30–60 minutes before bedtime.
c. Reserve for short-term use or special circumstances (e.g., jet lag).

Precaution:

- Not for children under age 3 unless prescribed.
- Avoid long-term use without medical guidance.
- May affect natural melatonin production if overused.

11. Room Temperature

Rationale:

Stable room temperature supports uninterrupted, safe sleep and prevents overheating or night waking.

Instructions:

a. Maintain a room temperature between 68–72°F (20–22°C).
b. Dress the child in breathable layers, typically one more than an adult would wear.
c. Use a fan or humidifier for air circulation in warm months
d. In cooler months, use a space heater with safety shut-off if needed, placed away from the sleep area.

Precaution:

- Avoid electric blankets and heating pads.
- Never place a crib or bed directly near vents, windows, or radiators.
- Watch for signs of overheating: sweating, flushed cheeks, or rapid breathing.
- Follow infant safe sleep guidelines for babies under 12 months.

12. Sleep Sacks and Wearable Blankets (Infants and Toddlers)

Rationale:

Wearable blankets help regulate temperature without the risk of suffocation. They support consistent sleep cues and are helpful during swaddle transitions.

Instructions:

a. Select a properly sized, sleeveless sleep sack for your child's age and development.

b. Use a TOG rating appropriate to the room temperature (0.5 TOG for warm rooms, 1.0–2.5 TOG for cooler environments).
c. Dress the child in breathable sleepwear underneath.
d. Ensure hips and legs can move freely.

Precaution:

- Do not use with swaddling once the child can roll over.
- Avoid overly thick sacks in warm climates.
- Monitor for signs of overheating.

13. Sound Machines and Gentle Music

Rationale:

Consistent background noise reduces startle responses and masks household disturbances, promoting deeper sleep.

Instructions:

a. Choose white noise, nature sounds, or soft lullabies.
b. Keep volume under 50 decibels.
c. Place the sound source at least several feet from the bed or crib.

14. Weighted Blankets (Age 3+ and Only When Appropriate)

Rationale:

Weighted blankets can calm the nervous system, improve body awareness, and promote better sleep—particularly for children with sensory sensitivities.

Instructions:

a. Select a blanket that is no more than 10% of the child's weight plus 1 pound.
b. Use only with children who can remove the blanket on their own.

c. Introduce during quiet time or bedtime routines before full overnight use.
d. Place the blanket over the torso or legs only, never the face.

Precaution:

- Do not use in children under age 3.
- Avoid use in children with respiratory or mobility issues unless cleared by a provider.
- Monitor closely for overheating or discomfort.

Daytime Habits That Impact Nighttime Sleep

Children's sleep quality is influenced not only by the bedtime routine but also by their daily habits, especially their diet and exposure to screens. The following strategies help support balanced rhythms throughout the day.

1. Limit Sugar and Processed Foods

Rationale:

High-sugar diets and foods containing artificial additives can contribute toc hyperactivity and poor sleep quality, particularly when consumed in the afternoon or evening.

Instructions:

a. Reduce intake of sugary snacks, sodas, and processed treats, especially in the hours leading up to bedtime.
b. Emphasize whole foods with healthy fats, proteins, and complex carbohydrates during dinner.
c. If sleep disruptions continue, consider eliminating artificial colors, sweeteners, and preservatives under the guidance of a healthcare provider.

2. Reduce Screen Time (Especially in the Evening)

Rationale:

Excessive screen use—particularly before bedtime—can suppress melatonin production and delay the body's natural sleep rhythm.

Instructions:

a. Limit total screen time for young children to 1–2 hours or less per day.
b. Turn off TVs, tablets, phones, and other screens at least 1–2 hours before bedtime.
c. Replace screens with calming evening routines such as reading, storytelling, or quiet play.

Night Terrors

Night terrors are episodes of intense fear, crying, or screaming during sleep, most common in children between the ages of 3 and 8. Unlike nightmares, night terrors occur during **non-REM (deep) sleep** and typically happen in the first third of the night. The child may appear awake—with open eyes and movement—but is not conscious and usually doesn't remember the event.

Signs and Symptoms:

- Sudden screaming, crying, or thrashing during sleep
- Rapid breathing or sweating
- Unresponsive to parental comfort
- Occurs early in the night, often within 1–2 hours of falling asleep
- No recollection of the event in the morning

When to Seek Immediate Medical Attention:

- Night terrors are frequent, prolonged, or causing safety concerns
- The child is excessively sleepy during the day
- Episodes include sleepwalking in unsafe environments
- There are signs of seizure-like activity
- Child has other signs of stress, trauma, or emotional distress

Comfort Measures and Natural Support for Night Terrors:

1. Emotional Support During the Day

Rationale:

Children experiencing stress, overstimulation, or emotional overload during the day may be more prone to night terrors.

Addressing emotional well-being can reduce their frequency and severity.

Instructions:

a. Encourage calm, grounding activities such as drawing, reading, quiet outdoor play, or nature walks.
b. Limit overstimulation from busy schedules, crowded environments, or excessive screen use.
c. Offer reassurance and comfort after each episode, even if the child has no memory of the event.

2. Ensure a Calm, Predictable Bedtime Routine

Rationale:

A consistent and soothing bedtime routine helps the nervous system settle and supports a smoother transition into deeper stages of sleep—where night terrors typically occur.

Instructions:

a. Avoid stimulating activities in the hour before bed (e.g., running, screens, intense games).
b. Follow the same pattern each evening (e.g., bath, book, music)
c. Keep sleep and wake times consistent, including week-ends.

3. Limit Screens and Sugar in the Evening

Rationale:

Evening exposure to screens and refined sugars can disrupt melatonin production and contribute to nervous system dys-regulation, increasing the likelihood of night terrors.

Instructions:

a. Avoid screen exposure for at least 1–2 hours before bedtime.

b. Limit sugary snacks, drinks, and processed foods in the afternoon and evening.
c. Offer calming snacks that include protein and healthy fats if the child is hungry before bed.

4. Support Deeper, Uninterrupted Sleep

Rationale:

Night terrors are more likely when sleep is fragmented or when a child is overtired. Creating an environment that supports uninterrupted, high-quality rest is essential.

Instructions:

a. Use white noise, blackout curtains, or a cool-mist humidifier to minimize disturbances.
b. Ensure your child is going to bed at an age-appropriate hour—overtiredness can be a common trigger.
c. Consider incorporating a warm magnesium bath before bed (see Sleep Support section, Remedy #9).

Sleep Regression

Sleep regression refers to a temporary disruption in sleep habits that occurs during specific stages of development. It may include increased night waking, difficulty falling asleep, or shortened naps. Common around **4 months**, **8–10 months**, **18 months**, and **2–3 years**, sleep regressions typically last 2–6 weeks.

Signs and Symptoms:

- Resistance to bedtime or nap time
- More frequent night wakings
- Fussiness or clinginess
- Sudden need for reassurance or night feeding
- Changes in appetite or behavior during the day

When to Seek Immediate Medical Attention:

- Sleep disruption is accompanied by signs of illness (fever, ear pain, cough, vomiting)
- Child stops gaining weight or refuses to eat
- Signs of anxiety, stress, or trauma are present
- Sleep disturbance persists for more than 6–8 weeks

Comfort Measures and Natural Strategies for Sleep Regression:

1. Encourage Daytime Activity and Outdoor Play

Rationale:

Physical movement and exposure to natural light during the day help regulate the circadian rhythm and support nighttime melatonin production, which may be disrupted during regressions.

Instructions:

a. Provide daily opportunities for outdoor play, movement, and sunlight exposure.

b. Adjust activity levels based on your child's age and energy needs.
c. Prevent overtiredness by observing wake windows and early sleep cues.

2. Maintain a Consistent Routine

Rationale:

Consistency reassures a child during developmental regressions and helps protect established sleep associations, preventing long-term sleep disruption.

Instructions:

a. Stick to regular bedtimes and nap times, even if sleep is temporarily disrupted.
b. Keep familiar pre-bedtime rituals such as bathing, reading, or music.
c. Avoid introducing new sleep habits (e.g., co-sleeping or late-night feedings) that may persist after the regression ends.

3. Offer Reassurance Without Reinforcing Wakefulness

Rationale:

Gentle reassurance helps soothe nighttime distress while avoiding habits that prolong wakefulness or delay independent sleep resettling.

Instructions:

a. Use soft words, calming touch, or quiet music to settle your child during night wakings.
b. Avoid turning on bright lights or fully waking the child unless necessary.
c. Gradually reduce involvement as the regression resolves to reestablish self-settling.

CHAPTER 12

ELIMINATING TOXINS

This section is for educational purposes only. The remedies listed are intended to support comfort and wellness and should not be used as a substitute for professional medical advice. Always consult your child's healthcare provider for diagnosis and treatment.

Eliminating Toxins in Childhood

As you read this section, remember that the goal is not perfection, but progress. Even small, gradual changes can impact your child's health and well-being over time.

Why Reducing Toxins Matters in Childhood

Children are uniquely vulnerable to environmental toxins due to their smaller size, rapidly developing organs, thinner skin, and frequent hand-to-mouth behavior. Their immature detoxification systems make it more difficult to eliminate harmful substances, increasing the risk of bioaccumulation over time.

Everyday exposures—from household cleaners, personal care products, food additives, plastics, air, water, and even clothing—can interfere with neurological development, hormonal balance, immune regulation, gut health, and sleep quality. These environmental toxins may quietly impact a child's long-term health and resilience.

Minimizing toxic exposures in the home is one of the most powerful and proactive ways to protect a child's well-being. This chapter offers evidence-informed, practical strategies for reducing common sources of toxicity and outlines gentle, age-appropriate detoxification support to help your child thrive in today's environment

Causes:

- Synthetic fragrances and chemical additives in personal care and cleaning products
- VOCs (volatile organic compounds) from air fresheners, paints, and plastics
- Flame retardants, pesticides, and heavy metals
- Plastic leaching from containers, toys, and cookware
- Processed foods with additives, dyes, and preservatives

- EMF (electromagnetic field) radiation from electronics and Wi-Fi

Signs & Symptoms:

In Infants & Toddlers:

- Skin irritation or rashes
- Breathing issues or chronic congestion
- Sleep disturbances
- Digestive upset or food sensitivities
- Behavioral changes or fussiness

Older Children May Experience:

- Headaches or fatigue
- Hormonal imbalances or early puberty signs
- Difficulty concentrating
- Allergies or recurrent infections
- Anxiety or sleep issues

1. Air Fresheners and Home Fragrances

Rationale:

Commercial air fresheners, scented candles, and sprays can emit volatile organic compounds (VOCs) and formaldehyde, which irritate the respiratory tract and disrupt hormone function.

Instructions:

a. Replace plug-ins, sprays, and synthetic candles with essential oil diffusers using diluted child-safe oils like lavender or citrus.
b. Simmer cinnamon sticks, orange peels, or herbs in water on the stove for a natural scent.
c. Freshen carpets with baking soda mixed with a few drops of essential oil—let sit 30 minutes, then vacuum.

Precaution:

- Do not use essential oils in infants under 6 months without provider guidance.
- Avoid eucalyptus and peppermint oils in children under 5.

2. Body Washes and Soaps

Rationale:

Children's skin is more permeable and sensitive than adult skin, allowing greater absorption of harmful chemicals like sulfates, parabens, and synthetic dyes.

Instructions:

a. Choose fragrance-free or naturally scented soaps made with simple, plant-based ingredients.
b. Look for castile soap, goat milk soap, or unscented olive oil–based cleansers.
c. Avoid bubble baths unless specifically labeled non-toxic and pediatric-safe

Precaution:

- Always patch test new soaps on a small area first.

3. Dish Soap and Bottle Cleaning

Rationale:

Residue from harsh dish soaps may remain on bottles and dishes, exposing children to synthetic preservatives and artificial fragrance.

Instructions:

a. Use food-safe, unscented, plant-based dish soaps.
b. Soak bottles or nipples in diluted white vinegar, then rinse thoroughly.

c. Avoid dish soaps with triclosan, sulfates, or artificial dyes.

Precaution:

- Rinse thoroughly after vinegar soaks to avoid taste irritation.

4. EMF and Wireless Exposure

Rationale:

Prolonged exposure to wireless radiation from routers, tablets, and cell phones may affect the developing nervous system and sleep patterns.

Instructions:

a. Unplug or turn off Wi-Fi routers at night, especially in sleeping areas.
b. Use airplane mode on tablets and phones during non-use.
c. For teens, place EMF-reducing phone sleeves on devices or encourage speakerphone use instead of holding to the head.
d. Keep devices away from the lap or body during use.

Precaution:

- Avoid EMF-blocking stickers with unverified claims—use tested shielding fabrics if needed.

5. Fertilizers and Bug Sprays

Rationale:

Many commercial lawn care products and insect repellents contain endocrine disruptors, neurotoxins, and carcinogens.

Instructions:

a. Opt for organic or child-safe lawn treatments.
b. Use neem oil, cedarwood, or essential-oil-based repellents.
c. Apply food-grade diatomaceous earth indoors for ant and flea control.

Precaution:

- Do not allow children to handle powdered products—apply and clean thoroughly afterward.

6. Food Quality and Additives

Rationale:

Artificial colors, sweeteners, preservatives, and pesticides in food may affect behavior, immunity, and long-term health.

Instructions:

a. Prioritize organic produce, especially those on the Dirty Dozen list (e.g., strawberries, spinach).
b. Soak fruits and vegetables in vinegar or baking soda and water before use.
c. Limit packaged snacks and cook with whole, unprocessed ingredients.

Precaution:

- Introduce dietary changes gradually to avoid food resistance.

7. Household Cleaning Products

Rationale:

Bleach, ammonia, and phenol-based products can irritate eyes, skin, and lungs, especially in enclosed spaces.

Instructions:

a. Use natural all-purpose spray: 1 cup vinegar + 1 cup water + 10 drops lemon or tea tree oil.
b. Make glass cleaner: 1 cup water + ½ cup vinegar + 1 tbsp rubbing alcohol.
c. For scrubbing paste: mix baking soda and castile soap to desired consistency.

Precaution:

- Never mix vinegar with bleach or ammonia.
- Keep all cleaning products locked away from children.

8. Laundry Products

Homemade Laundry Detergent

Rationale:

Conventional laundry detergents often contain optical brighteners, artificial fragrance, and hormone-disrupting preservatives.

Instructions:

a. Choose fragrance-free, plant-based detergents labeled "non-toxic" or "free and clear."
b. Always wash new clothing before wear.
c. Homemade laundry detergent:

- 1 cup washing soda
- 1 cup baking soda
- 1 bar grated castile soap
- 10 drops lavender oil (optional)

Use 2–3 tbsp per load.

Using Wool Dryer Balls with Essential Oils

Rationale:

Wool dryer balls naturally soften clothing, reduce static, and shorten drying time without the use of synthetic fragrances or chemicals. Adding essential oils provides a light, natural scent without exposing children to endocrine-disrupting compounds found in conventional dryer sheets.

Instructions:

a. Place 3–6 wool dryer balls into the dryer with your wet laundry.
b. Add 2–3 drops of a child-safe essential oil (such as **lavender** or **chamomile**) to each ball.
c. Let the oil absorb for a few minutes before placing in the dryer to avoid oil stains.
d. Run the dryer on a low or medium heat setting as usual.
e. Reapply essential oil every few loads as needed.

Precaution:

- Use only essential oils that are safe for children and properly diluted.
- Do not use peppermint, eucalyptus, or rosemary oils for children under 6 years.
- Ensure dryer balls are fully dry between uses to prevent mildew.

9. Lotions and Moisturizers

Rationale:

Many store-bought lotions contain petroleum, synthetic fragrance, and hormone disruptors that can be absorbed through the skin.

Instructions:

a. Use simple moisturizers like coconut oil, olive oil, tallow, or shea butter.
b. Breast milk can be applied topically for infants with skin irritation.
c. Choose products with full ingredient disclosure.

Precaution:

- Avoid mineral oil, PEGs, and anything labeled "fragrance."

10. Makeup and Skincare (Tweens and Teens)

Rationale:

Many tween-targeted makeup and skincare products contain parabens, phthalates, and synthetic fragrance. Establishing safe habits early protects hormonal and skin health.

Instructions:

a. Choose clean brands with EWG-verified ingredients or third-party certifications.
b. Look for mineral-based powders and tinted balms over foundation and lipstick.
c. Use simple moisturizers and cleansers made with calendula, aloe, or tea tree for acne-prone skin.

Precaution:

- Avoid products with glitter, artificial fragrance, and dyes.
- Educate tweens on reading labels and patch-testing new products.

11. Perfumes and Fragrance Oils

Rationale:

Synthetic fragrances often contain phthalates and hidden chemical ingredients that can interfere with endocrine function.

Instructions:

a. Use diluted essential oil rollers (e.g., lavender or orange) for older children and teens.
b. Diffuse calming oils before bedtime using a cool-mist diffuser.

Precaution:

- Do not apply essential oils directly to young children's skin.
- Avoid perfume sprays entirely for children under age 10.

12. Plastics, Cookware, and Food Storage

Rationale:

Plastics can leach BPA, phthalates, or microplastics, especially when heated, affecting hormonal balance.

Instructions:

a. Use stainless steel or glass for water bottles and food storage.
b. Replace nonstick and aluminum pans with cast iron or ceramic-coated options.
c. Never microwave plastic containers.

Precaution:

- Discard scratched plastic items, which leach more chemicals.

13. Toys and School Supplies

Rationale:

Toys, art supplies, and school items can contain PVC, formaldehyde, and lead, especially when imported or unlabeled.

Instructions:

a. Choose toys made of wood, silicone, or organic cotton.
b. Use beeswax crayons and non-toxic glue and paint.
c. Avoid scented markers or glitter glue.

Precaution:

- Always supervise younger children with craft materials.

14. Water Quality

Rationale:

Tap water can contain lead, fluoride, chlorine, nitrates, and microplastics that burden the body over time.

Instructions:

a. Install a high-quality water filter for drinking and cooking.
b. Use filtered showerheads or bath filters, especially for children with skin sensitivities.
c. Choose glass or stainless-steel water bottles.

Precaution:

- Change filters according to manufacturer guidelines to prevent bacterial buildup

Gentle Detox Methods for Children

Before beginning any oral or topical detox method, always consult a pediatric healthcare provider. Detoxification in children should be gentle, short-term, and carefully supervised.

Bath Safety Reminder:

Never leave children unattended in the bath. Always test water temperature and patch test any oils or new ingredients.

1. Detox Baths

Warm detox baths support circulation, lymph flow, and gentle elimination.

Ingredients:

- Epsom salt (½ cup)
- Baking soda (¼ cup)
- Bentonite clay (1–2 tbsp, premixed)
- Child-safe essential oils (1–2 drops in carrier oil)

Instructions:

a. Add chosen ingredients to warm water
b. Soak for 15–20 minutes
c. Rinse thoroughly after bath

Oral Detox Supports for Children

With Pediatric Guidance Only

These gentle oral remedies may support the body's natural detoxification processes by assisting the liver, lymphatic system, gastrointestinal tract, and cellular cleansing. Use only age-appropriate products and consult your pediatrician before use—especially if your child has allergies, chronic conditions, or is on medication.

1. Aloe Vera Juice (Inner Fillet Only)

Rationale:

Aloe vera supports digestion, soothes the gut lining, and promotes gentle elimination. It can assist the detox process by reducing inflammation in the gastrointestinal tract and improving bowel regularity.

Instructions:

a. Use only organic, decolorized inner fillet aloe juice (free from aloin).
b. For children over age 3, begin with 1–2 teaspoons diluted in water or juice once daily.
c. Offer on an empty stomach or before meals.

Precaution:

- Not for children under 2.
- Avoid use if your child has diarrhea or loose stools, as it may worsen symptoms.

2. Apple Cider Vinegar (ACV)

Rationale:

Raw apple cider vinegar supports digestion, promotes healthy gut bacteria, and may help the body maintain an optimal pH balance. It assists gentle detoxification by encouraging liver and lymphatic function.

Instructions:

a. Dilute 1 teaspoon of raw, unfiltered ACV in a small glass of warm water.
b. Add a small amount of raw honey (for children over 1 year) to improve taste.
c. Offer once daily, preferably before meals.

Precaution:

- Never serve undiluted ACV—it can irritate the throat and damage tooth enamel.
- Use a straw to reduce contact with teeth, and rinse the mouth afterward.

3. Cod Liver Oil

Rationale:

Cod liver oil is rich in omega-3 fatty acids (EPA and DHA) and natural vitamins A and D, which support liver function, reduce inflammation, and promote immune regulation. It is especially beneficial during or after illness and as part of a gentle detox strategy.

Instructions:

a. Choose a purified, third-party tested cod liver oil formulated for children.
b. Administer according to age-specific dosage on the label or as advised by your provider.
c. Mix with juice, applesauce, or a smoothie to reduce taste aversion.

Precaution:

- Do not exceed the recommended dosage to avoid excess vitamin A.

- Avoid combining with other high-dose vitamin A or D supplements unless directed by a healthcare provider.

4. Dandelion Root Tea (Ages 5+)

Rationale:

Dandelion root gently stimulates liver and kidney function, helping the body filter and excrete toxins. It also acts as a mild diuretic to support lymphatic drainage.

Instructions:

a. Steep 1 teaspoon of dried dandelion root in 1 cup of hot water for 5–10 minutes.
b. Cool completely and offer 2–4 tablespoons to children over age 5.
c. Use up to once daily during short periods of detox support.

Precaution:

- Do not use in children with gallbladder disorders or known plant allergies.
- Monitor closely for allergic reactions after the first dose.

5. Fulvic Acid (Liquid Trace Minerals)

Rationale:

Fulvic acid enhances nutrient absorption and helps chelate (bind and remove) toxins, including glyphosate and heavy metals. It also supports cellular energy and immune function.

Instructions:

a. Use trace mineral drops or fulvic acid supplements designed for children.
b. Mix the recommended dose into filtered water or juice once daily.

c. Offer alongside food for improved absorption.

Precaution:

- Avoid overuse, especially in infants and toddlers.
- Use only trace amounts and discontinue use if digestive changes or fatigue occur.

6. Glutathione (Liposomal or Oral Spray)

Rationale:

Glutathione is the body's master antioxidant, essential for cellular detoxification, liver function, and immune regulation. Supplementing with glutathione may enhance the body's ability to neutralize and eliminate toxins.

Instructions:

a. Use only pediatric-formulated glutathione (liposomal liquid or spray).
b. Follow the age-based dosing instructions provided on the product label.
c. Administer on an empty stomach or between meals for optimal absorption.

Precaution:

- Use only under pediatric supervision.
- Not recommended for daily long-term use unless directed by a provider.
- Discontinue if rash or digestive upset occurs.

7. Liquid Chlorophyll

Rationale:

Chlorophyll, a plant pigment, supports cellular detox by binding to toxins and heavy metals. It also enhances oxygenation and helps neutralize internal acidity and odor.

Instructions:

a. Use food-grade liquid chlorophyll designed for children.
b. Begin with 5–10 drops mixed into water or juice once daily.
c. Gradually increase as tolerated, if recommended by your provider.

Precaution:

- May cause temporary dark green stools.
- Discontinue if digestive upset occurs.
- Avoid in children with sensitivity to algae or green superfoods.

8. Spirulina or Chlorella

Rationale:

These nutrient-rich algae support detoxification by binding to heavy metals and providing essential minerals, antioxidants, and B vitamins. They promote gut health and immune resilience.

Instructions:

a. Choose certified organic, third-party tested spirulina or chlorella powder.
b. Mix a small amount (⅛ to ¼ teaspoon) into smoothies, applesauce, or juice for older children.
c. Use 1–3 times per week as part of a rotating supplement plan.

Precaution:

d. May cause digestive upset in sensitive children or those with iodine issues.
e. Avoid if your child has an autoimmune condition without provider guidance.

9. Zeolite (Clinoptilolite)

Rationale:

Zeolite is a naturally occurring volcanic mineral that helps trap and eliminate heavy metals and environmental toxins from the digestive tract. It supports detox without being absorbed systemically.

Instructions:

a. Use only purified, micronized zeolite labeled safe for children.
b. Mix the recommended dose (typically a few drops or powder) into water or juice.
c. Use 2–3 times per week during targeted detox periods.

Precaution:

- Ensure your child stays hydrated while using zeolite, as it may bind to minerals.
- Avoid combining with medications or other supplements without provider input.

Gut Health and Daily Detox Support

A healthy gut supports detoxification through regular bowel movements, immune defense, and toxin binding.

Supportive Strategies:

- Use high-quality probiotics with appropriate strains
- Offer prebiotic foods like bananas, garlic, oats
- Avoid processed sugar and dyes
- Include bone broth, fiber, and hydration daily
- Promote daily elimination through movement and diet

Daily Home Detox Checklist

- Use fragrance-free laundry and dish soap
- Eliminate air fresheners, candles, and scent beads
- Filter drinking and bathing water
- Avoid plastics in cookware and food storage
- Vacuum regularly with a HEPA filter
- Open windows daily for fresh air
- Use non-toxic cleaning products
- Prioritize whole, organic foods
- Support regular bowel movements
- Spend time outside and reduce screen exposure
- Diffuse essential oils instead of using synthetic scents
- Limit EMF exposure during sleep

DISCLAIMER

Terezia Tarantino is a Doctor of Nursing Practice, not a medical doctor. The information in this book is intended for **informational and educational purposes only** on the topic of supplemental and comfort care. **It is not intended to replace traditional care, diagnosis, or treatment of medical conditions**. The remedies and practices discussed should complement professional medical care and are not a substitute.

Before using any remedies or implementing the suggestions provided, it is essential to consult with your trusted pediatric, primary care provider, or healthcare professional to ensure they are appropriate for your child's specific needs and health conditions. Individual responses to treatments and remedies can vary, and professional guidance is essential for making informed decisions.

In the event of a medical emergency or if your child experiences severe symptoms, please seek **immediate** medical attention by calling 911 or visiting your nearest emergency care facility. Always prioritize professional medical care and follow the advice of your healthcare provider, particularly for severe or urgent health concerns.

The author and publisher disclaim any liability for adverse effects or consequences resulting from the use or misuse of the information contained in this book. By utilizing this resource, you acknowledge that you are solely responsible for the health and well-being of your child and that this book is

NOT intended to replace medical advice or care from your licensed healthcare professionals.

Home remedies are **NOT** appropriate during instances of extremely high fevers (Those over 104), difficulty breathing, trauma (serious injury to the head, skeletal system, or deep wounds), or ingestion of poisonous or unknown substances. Always seek professional medical attention if in doubt

REFERENCES

Chapter 1: Ears

1. American Academy of Pediatrics. (2023). *Ear infections in children.* https://www.healthychildren.org
2. Mayo Clinic. (2023). *Ear infection (middle ear).* https://www.mayoclinic.org/diseases-conditions/ear-infections
3. National Institutes of Health. (2022). *Otitis media overview.* https://www.ncbi.nlm.nih.gov
4. WebMD. (2023). *Earwax blockage and removal.* https://www.webmd.com
5. Tisserand, R., & Young, R. (2014). *Essential oil safety: A guide for health care professionals* (2nd ed.). Churchill Livingstone.
6. Gladstar, R. (2008). *Herbal recipes for vibrant health.* Storey Publishing.
7. Natural Medicines Database. (2024). *Tea tree oil (Melaleuca alternifolia) monograph.*
8. National Center for Complementary and Integrative Health. (2023). *Garlic.* https://www.nccih.nih.gov/health/garlic
9. American Academy of Otolaryngology–Head and Neck Surgery. (2023). *Swimmer's ear (otitis externa).* https://www.entnet.org

Chapter 2: Nose

1. Centers for Disease Control and Prevention. (2023). *Common colds: Protect yourself and others.* https://www.cdc.gov
2. Mayo Clinic. (2023). *Sinusitis.* https://www.mayoclinic.org
3. American Academy of Pediatrics. (2023). *Nasal congestion in infants and children.* https://www.healthychildren.org
4. National Center for Complementary and Integrative Health. (2023). *Eucalyptus.* https://www.nccih.nih.gov
5. Tisserand, R., & Young, R. (2014). *Essential oil safety* (2nd ed.).
6. University of Maryland Medical Center. (2023). *Nasal saline irrigation (Neti pot).*
7. WebMD. (2023). *Nasal polyps and chronic congestion.* https://www.webmd.com
8. American College of Allergy, Asthma, and Immunology. (2023). *Allergic rhinitis.* https://acaai.org

Chapter 3: Mouth and Throat

1. Mayo Clinic. (2023). *Oral thrush in children.* https://www.mayoclinic.org
2. Cleveland Clinic. (2023). *Strep throat.* https://my.clevelandclinic.org
3. Centers for Disease Control and Prevention. (2023). *Hand, foot, and mouth disease (HFMD).* https://www.cdc.gov
4. WebMD. (2023). *Teething symptoms and remedies.* https://www.webmd.com
5. National Center for Complementary and Integrative Health. (2023). *Chamomile.* https://www.nccih.nih.gov
6. Tisserand, R., & Young, R. (2014). *Essential oil safety* (2nd ed.).

7. Herbal Safety. (n.d.). *Calendula (Calendula officinalis).* University of Texas at El Paso and University of Texas–Austin Cooperative.
8. Natural Medicines Database. (2024). *Grapefruit seed extract monograph.*
9. Weil, A. (2022). *Dr. Weil's natural remedies for sore throat and teething.* https://www.drweil.com

Chapter 4: Eyes and Head

1. American Academy of Ophthalmology. (2022). *Conjunctivitis (pink eye).* https://www.aao.org
2. Mayo Clinic. (2023). *Stye.* https://www.mayoclinic.org
3. Mayo Clinic. (2023). *Chalazion.* https://www.mayoclinic.org
4. Mayo Clinic. (2023). *Foreign object in the eye: First aid.* https://www.mayoclinic.org
5. Centers for Disease Control and Prevention. (2023). *Head lice.* https://www.cdc.gov/parasites/lice/head/index.html
6. American Academy of Dermatology Association. (2023). *Dandruff: Diagnosis and treatment.* https://www.aad.org
7. National Headache Foundation. (2023). *Types of headaches in children.* https://headaches.org
8. National Center for Complementary and Integrative Health. (2023). *Chamomile.* https://www.nccih.nih.gov
9. Natural Medicines Database. (2024). *Tea tree oil (Melaleuca alternifolia) monograph.*
10. Tisserand, R., & Young, R. (2014). *Essential oil safety* (2nd ed.).
11. Weil, A. (2022). *Dr. Weil's Guide to Optimum Health.* https://www.drweil.com

Chapter 5: Respiratory System

1. American Academy of Pediatrics. (2023). *Signs of breathing problems in children.* https://www.healthychildren.org
2. Centers for Disease Control and Prevention. (2023). *Honey and infant botulism.* https://www.cdc.gov
3. National Institutes of Health. (2022). *Manuka honey: Antibacterial and wound-healing properties.* https://www.ncbi.nlm.nih.gov/pmc/articles/PMC3609166/
4. National Center for Complementary and Integrative Health. (2023). *Eucalyptus.* https://www.nccih.nih.gov
5. National Center for Complementary and Integrative Health. (2023). *Ginger.* https://www.nccih.nih.gov
6. National Center for Complementary and Integrative Health. (2023). *Chamomile.* https://www.nccih.nih.gov
7. University of Maryland Medical Center. (2022). *Mullein (Verbascum thapsus).*
8. Tisserand, R., & Young, R. (2014). *Essential oil safety* (2nd ed.).
9. Gladstar, R. (2008). *Herbal recipes for vibrant health.* Storey Publishing.
10. Buhner, S. H. (2012). *Herbal antibiotics* (2nd ed.). Storey Publishing.
11. American Lung Association. (2023). *Breathing exercises for children.* https://www.lung.org
12. National Jewish Health. (2023). *Chest physical therapy (CPT) for children.* https://www.nationaljewish.org
13. Environmental Protection Agency. (2023). *Using humidifiers safely.* https://www.epa.gov

Chapter 6: Gastrointestinal Health

1. Centers for Disease Control and Prevention. (2023). *Dehydration and children*. https://www.cdc.gov
2. Mayo Clinic. (2023). *Diarrhea*. https://www.mayoclinic.org
3. Mayo Clinic. (2023). *Constipation in children*. https://www.mayoclinic.org
4. National Center for Complementary and Integrative Health. (2023). *Ginger*. https://www.nccih.nih.gov
5. National Center for Complementary and Integrative Health. (2023). *Chamomile*. https://www.nccih.nih.gov
6. Herbal Safety. (n.d.). *Marshmallow root*. University of Texas at El Paso and University of Texas–Austin Cooperative. https://www.herbalsafety.utep.edu
7. Natural Medicines Database. (2024). *Grapefruit seed extract monograph*.
8. Natural Medicines Database. (2024). *Slippery elm monograph*.
9. Tisserand, R., & Young, R. (2014). *Essential oil safety: A guide for health care professionals* (2nd ed.). Churchill Livingstone.
10. Gladstar, R. (2008). *Herbal recipes for vibrant health*. Storey Publishing.
11. American Academy of Pediatrics. (2023). *Managing vomiting and diarrhea in children*. https://www.healthychildren.org
12. Weil, A. (2022). *Dr. Weil's natural health tips*. https://www.drweil.com
13. WebMD. (2023). *Constipation in infants and children*. https://www.webmd.com
14. Harvard Health Publishing. (2023). *Probiotics and the gut*. https://www.health.harvard.edu

15. Academy of Nutrition and Dietetics. (2023). *Nutrition for children with gastrointestinal conditions*. https://www.eat-right.org
16. Environmental Protection Agency. (2023). *Safe drinking water*. https://www.epa.gov

Chapter 7: Urinary Health

1. Mayo Clinic. (2023). *Urinary tract infection (UTI) in children*. https://www.mayoclinic.org
2. Centers for Disease Control and Prevention. (2023). *Urinary tract infections*. https://www.cdc.gov
3. American Academy of Pediatrics. (2023). *Urinary problems in children*. https://www.healthychildren.org
4. National Institutes of Health. (2022). *Dysuria and other urinary symptoms in pediatrics*. https://www.ncbi.nlm.nih.gov
5. Harvard Health Publishing. (2023). *Cranberry juice and urinary tract infections*. https://www.health.harvard.edu
6. Natural Medicines Database. (2024). *Cranberry monograph*.
7. National Center for Complementary and Integrative Health. (2023). *Chamomile*. https://www.nccih.nih.gov
8. Herbal Safety. (n.d.). *Marshmallow root*. University of Texas at El Paso and University of Texas–Austin Cooperative. https://www.herbalsafety.utep.edu
9. Tisserand, R., & Young, R. (2014). *Essential oil safety: A guide for health care professionals* (2nd ed.). Churchill Livingstone.
10. WebMD. (2023). *Painful urination in children*. https://www.webmd.com
11. Cleveland Clinic. (2023). *Daytime wetting and urinary retention in children*. https://my.clevelandclinic.org

12. National Institute of Diabetes and Digestive and Kidney Diseases. (2023). *Bedwetting (nocturnal enuresis).* https://www.niddk.nih.gov
13. American Urological Association. (2023). *Pediatric voiding dysfunction and urinary incontinence.* https://www.auanet.org
14. National Center for Complementary and Integrative Health. (2023). *Lemon balm.* https://www.nccih.nih.gov
15. Academy of Nutrition and Dietetics. (2023). *Hydration and urinary health in children.* https://www.eatright.org

Chapter 8 Skin Health

1. American Academy of Dermatology Association. (n.d.). *Diaper rash: Tips for preventing and treating.* https://www.aad.org
2. Mayo Clinic. (2022). *Eczema (atopic dermatitis).* https://www.mayoclinic.org
3. National Eczema Association. (n.d.). *Eczema treatments and relief.* https://nationaleczema.org
4. Levy, M. L., & Sheikh, A. (2015). *Managing childhood eczema: A practical guide.* BMJ, 350, h1580. https://doi.org/10.1136/bmj.h1580
5. Healthline. (2023). *Home remedies for heat rash in babies and toddlers.* https://www.healthline.com
6. WebMD. (2021). *Contact dermatitis in children.* https://www.webmd.com/skin-problems-and-treatments/guide/irritant-contact-dermatitis
7. Centers for Disease Control and Prevention. (2022). *Impetigo: For healthcare professionals.* https://www.cdc.gov/
8. Bingham, A. (2021). *Natural remedies for impetigo: What works?.* Journal of Integrative Dermatology, 6(3), 122–127.

9. American Academy of Pediatrics. (n.d.). *Molluscum contagiosum: Advice for parents.* https://www.healthychildren.org

10. National Institutes of Health. (2020). *Apple cider vinegar as a topical treatment: A review.* Complementary Therapies in Medicine, 51, 102427. https://doi.org/10.1016/j.ctim.2020.102427

11. Cleveland Clinic. (2023). *Ringworm (tinea corporis): Causes, symptoms, and treatment.* https://my.clevelandclinic.org

12. Mays, J. W., & Aronson, I. K. (2021). *Pediatric dermatophytosis: Diagnosis and management.* Pediatric Clinics of North America, 68(5), 1025–1041.

13. American College of Emergency Physicians. (n.d.). *Burns: First aid and home care.* https://www.emergencyphysicians.org

14. Natural Medicine Journal. (2020). *Honey in wound healing: A review of clinical efficacy and mechanisms.* https://www.naturalmedicinejournal.com

15. Sovereign Silver. (n.d.). *Benefits of colloidal silver for skin healing.* https://www.sovereignsilver.com

16. Skin Cancer Foundation. (2023). *Sunburn: Risks and treatments in children.* https://www.skincancer.org

17. U.S. National Library of Medicine. (2021). *Managing sunburn in children: A guide for caregivers.* MedlinePlus. https://medlineplus.gov

18. American Academy of Allergy, Asthma & Immunology. (2022). *Insect sting reactions.* https://www.aaaai.org

19. National Institutes of Health. (2019). *Jellyfish stings: Evaluation and treatment.* https://www.ncbi.nlm.nih.gov/books/NBK537115/

20. Herbal Medicine Compendium. (2020). *Plant-based remedies for insect bites and stings in pediatrics.* Integrative Pediatrics Review, 12(2), 95–103.

Chapter 9 Fever

1. American Academy of Pediatrics. (2023). *Fever in children: When to worry, what to do.* https://www.healthychildren.org
2. Mayo Clinic. (2022). *Fever in children.* https://www.mayoclinic.org
3. Cleveland Clinic. (2021). *Febrile seizures: Causes, symptoms, and treatment.* https://my.clevelandclinic.org
4. National Institutes of Health. (2020). *Febrile seizures.* MedlinePlus. https://medlineplus.gov
5. Healthline. (2023). *Home remedies for fever in toddlers and children.* https://www.healthline.com
6. Natural Medicine Journal. (2019). *Herbal support for pediatric fevers: An integrative approach.* https://www.naturalmedicinejournal.com
7. WebMD. (2021). *What to do if your child has a fever.* https://www.webmd.com
8. National Center for Complementary and Integrative Health. (2022). *Peppermint oil and herbal remedies: Safety in children.* https://www.nccih.nih.gov
9. Aviva Romm, M.D. (2017). *Botanical medicine for children's fevers and infections.* https://avivaromm.com
10. Blatteis, C. M. (2012). *Fever: Pathogenesis and implications for treatment.* Annals of the New York Academy of Sciences, 1262(1), 1–6. https://doi.org/10.1111/j.1749-6632.2012.06672.x

Chapter 10 Immune Support

1. Munchkin Time. (2023). *Ginger Lemon Honey Syrup Recipe (Natural Immune Booster).* Retrieved from https://www.munchkintime.com/ginger-lemon-honey-syrup-recipe-natural-immune-booster/Munchkin Time

2. Wilder Child. (2014). *Flu Blasting, Kid-Approved Elderberry Syrup Recipe.* Retrieved from https://wilderchild.com/blogs/news/elderberry-syrup-recipewilderchild.com
3. Fare Isle. (2020). *Fire Cider Recipe for Immune Support.* Retrieved from https://fareisle.com/fire-cider/Fare Isle
4. New York Post. (2025). *My recipe for 'Amish amoxicillin' is all natural - it's the remedy we tried before going to the doctor.* Retrieved from https://nypost.com/2025/01/03/health/amish-amoxicillin-recipe-used-to-treat-illness-before-doctor/New York Post+1Flipboard+1
5. Sovereign Silver. (n.d.). *Bio-Active Silver Hydrosol for Kids | Spray | 4+ y.o.* Retrieved from https://www.amazon.com/Sovereign-Silver%C2%AE-Bio-Active-Silver-HydrosolTM/dp/B0716BTCYVTarget+2Amazon+2Chiro For Moms+2
6. Zicam. (n.d.). *Cold Remedy Homeopathic Nasal Swabs.* Retrieved from https://www.zicam.com/our-products/cold-shortening/nasal-swabsWalmart.com+3Zicam.com+3Amazon+3
7. Children's Health of Orange County (CHOC). (2023). *8 Superfoods to Boost Your Child's Diet.* Retrieved from https://health.choc.org/8-superfoods-to-boost-your-childs-diet/CHOC - Children's health hub
8. Children's Hospital of Philadelphia (CHOP). (2021). *Vitamin D Supplements: What Parents Should Know.* Retrieved from https://www.chop.edu/news/health-tip/vitamin-d-supplements-what-parents-should-knowChildren's Health+2Children's Hospital of Philadelphia+2Children's Hospital of Philadelphia+2
9. Run Wild My Child. (2023). *Grounding with Kids - The Benefits of Earthing for Kids.* Retrieved from https://runwildmychild.com/?p=11109RUN WILD MY CHILD+1Grooni Earthing+1
10. Children's Hospital of Philadelphia (CHOP). (2021). *Aromatherapy for Children: What's Safe and What's Not.* Retrieved from https://www.chop.edu/news/health-tip/

aromatherapy-children-whats-safe-and-whats-notChildren's Hospital of Philadelphia+1Children's Hospital of Philadelphia+1

Chapter 11: Sleep Support

1. American Academy of Pediatrics. (2021). *Healthy sleep habits: How many hours does your child need?* Retrieved from https://www.healthychildren.org/English/healthy-living/sleep/Pages/Healthy-Sleep-Habits-How-Many-Hours-Does-Your-Child-Need.aspx
2. National Sleep Foundation. (n.d.). *Children and sleep.* Retrieved from https://www.sleepfoundation.org/children-and-sleep
3. Centers for Disease Control and Prevention. (2020). *How much sleep do I need?* Retrieved from https://www.cdc.gov/sleep/about_sleep/how_much_sleep.html
4. KidsHealth from Nemours. (n.d.). *Night terrors.* Retrieved from https://kidshealth.org/en/parents/terrors.html
5. Healthline. (2022). *Night terrors in toddlers: Causes, management, and prevention.* Retrieved from https://www.healthline.com/health/night-terrors-in-toddlers
6. Children's Hospital of Philadelphia. (n.d.). *Helping your child cope with night terrors.* Retrieved from https://www.chop.edu/news/health-tip/more-just-bad-dream-helping-your-child-cope-night-terrors
7. Verywell Family. (2023). *What are toddler night terrors?* Retrieved from https://www.verywellfamily.com/what-to-do-about-infant-night-terrors-4174298
8. Natural Grocers. (n.d.). *Helping your little (and not so little) ones get a good night's sleep.* Retrieved from https://www.naturalgrocers.com/article/helping-your-little-and-not-so-little-ones-get-good-nights-sleep
9. Toronto Kids Health. (2023). *A parent's guide to safe herbal teas for children who have trouble falling asleep.* Retrieved

from https://www.torontokidshealth.com/a-parent-s-guide-to-safe-herbal-teas-for-children-who-have-trouble-falling-asleep

10. Thrive Family Chiropractic. (2023). *Natural sleep remedies for kids.* Retrieved from https://www.thrivefamchiropractic.com/natural-sleep-remedies-for-kids/
11. PX Docs. (2023). *Natural sleep remedies for kids.* Retrieved from https://pxdocs.com/natural-remedies/natural-sleep-remedies-for-kids/

Chapter 12 Eliminating Toxins

1. Centers for Disease Control and Prevention (CDC). (n.d.). *Principles of Pediatric Environmental Health: Why Are Children Especially Vulnerable to Environmental Toxicants?* Agency for Toxic Substances and Disease Registry. Retrieved from https://archive.cdc.gov/www_atsdr_cdc_gov/csem/pediatric-environmental-health/why_children.htmlCDC Archive
2. University of Arkansas Division of Agriculture. (n.d.). *Clean and Green Homemade Cleaners.* Retrieved from https://www.uaex.uada.edu/environment-nature/water/quality/clean-green-homemade-cleaners.aspxArkansas Cooperative Extension
3. HealthyChildren.org. (2024). *Green Cleaning: Choosing Products That Are Safer for Your Family.* American Academy of Pediatrics. Retrieved from https://www.healthychildren.org/English/safety-prevention/all-around/Pages/green-cleaning-choosing-products-that-are-safer-for-your-family.aspxHealthyChildren.org
4. Environmental Health Sciences Center, UC Davis. (2022). *Are Environmental Toxins Haunting Our Kids?* Retrieved from https://environmentalhealth.ucdavis.edu/blog/children-environmental-health-monthUCD Environmental Health Center

5. Boulder Holistic Functional Medicine. (2024). *10 Surprising Ways To Safely Detox Your Kids' Lives*. Retrieved from https://boulderholistic.com/10-surprising-ways-to-safely-detox-your-kids-lives/Boulder Holistic
6. Whole Child Texas. (2024). *Top 7 Tips to Detoxify Children Safely and Naturally*. Retrieved from https://www.wholechildtexas.com/blog/top-7-tips-to-detoxify-children-safely-and-naturally/wholechildtexas.com
7. Dr. Green Mom. (2022). *10 Ways To Support Detoxification In Kids*. Retrieved from https://drgreenmom.com/10-ways-to-support-detoxification-in-kids/Dr. Green Mom
8. Centers for Disease Control and Prevention (CDC). (n.d.). *Children's Environmental Health: Chemicals of Special Concern*. Minnesota Department of Health. Retrieved from https://www.health.state.mn.us/communities/environment/childenvhealth/chemicals.htmlMN Dept. of Health
9. Environmental Protection Agency (EPA). (2024). *Our Current Understanding of the Human Health and Environmental Risks of PFAS*. Retrieved from https://www.epa.gov/pfas/our-current-understanding-human-health-and-environmental-risks-pfasUS EPA
10. Wikipedia contributors. (2025). *Lead poisoning*. Wikipedia. Retrieved from https://en.wikipedia.org/wiki/Lead_poisoningWikipedia
11. Wikipedia contributors. (2025). *Chlorpyrifos*. Wikipedia. Retrieved from https://en.wikipedia.org/wiki/ChlorpyrifosWikipedia
12. Wikipedia contributors. (2025). *Plastic pollution*. Wikipedia. Retrieved from https://en.wikipedia.org/wiki/Plastic_pollution
13. Wikipedia contributors. (2025). *Health effects of pesticides*. Wikipedia. Retrieved from https://en.wikipedia.org/wiki/Health_effects_of_pesticides

14. Wikipedia contributors. (2025). *Endocrine disruptor*. Wikipedia. Retrieved from https://en.wikipedia.org/wiki/Endocrine_disruptor

15. Centers for Disease Control and Prevention (CDC). (n.d.). *Pediatric Chemical Exposure: Opportunities for Prevention*. Retrieved from https://www.sciencedirect.com/science/article/abs/pii/S0891524521002194ScienceDirect

16. The Good Trade. (2025). *10 Best Natural And Nontoxic Cleaning Products*. Retrieved from https://www.thegoodtrade.com/features/natural-nontoxic-cleaning-products/The Good Trade

17. Branch Basics. (n.d.). *Human Safe Cleaning Products*. Retrieved from https://branchbasics.com/Boulder Holistic+6Branch Basics+6The Good Trade+6

18. Blueland. (n.d.). *Eco-Friendly Cleaning Products for Home*. Retrieved from https://www.blueland.com/blueland.com

19. Healthy Kids Happy Kids. (2018). *Top 10 Ways to Safely Detox Your Child*. Retrieved from https://healthykidshappykids.com/2018/07/22/top-10-ways-safely-detox-child/Healthy Kids Happy Kids

20. CentreSpringMD. (2017). *Gentle Detox for Kids*. Retrieved from https://centrespringmd.com/gentle-detox-kids/CentreSpring MD

www.ingramcontent.com/pod-product-compliance
Lightning Source LLC
LaVergne TN
LVHW052028200926
848481LV00005B/1615
* 9 7 9 8 8 6 8 9 7 0 0 5 4 *